TRUE BLOOD NEVER LIES

Novel

NINO S. THEVENY

Self-published

Translated from French to English

By Jacquie Bridonneau

Original Title : *Trouble Je*

Created with Vellum

For

Nino and Luce, two little seeds who grew while this book was in gestation…

Prologue

The man sporting a ponytail unintentionally gripped his fingers on the cold steering wheel and clenched his jaw. His entire body was aiming for the same goal: exorcizing his old demons. Finally putting an end to so many long years of accumulated bitterness, pain and hatred.

He took another sip from the miniature bottle he'd purchased on the way, to warm him up and give him one last ounce of liquid courage.

Then he stepped on the gas.

The vehicle picked up speed, screeching, going through the intersection at the same time as another car.

The shock was brutal, inexorable and undoubtedly fatal...

Had his window been open, a passerby could have heard him shouting

"Revenge!" a second before the crash.

Part I

Chapter 1

Paris, October 2005

THE CONCORDE LAFAYETTE'S panoramic bar was the favorite watering hole for congress attendees at the Porte-Maillot Palais events.

Seated at a table overlooking the Bois de Boulogne park, Professor Siethbüller was enjoying a glass of champagne with his Gabonese colleague, Professor Francois N'Gapet, from Lambarene Hospital.

"My dear Francois, I'm so happy you could come to Paris this year after all this time! Cheers, my dear friend!"

"And I wish you good health, happiness, and prosperity," replied Professor N'Gapet. "What a beautiful place! A magnificent view and a superb hotel."

"I know, I've always liked to come here to enjoy a drink with my colleagues."

"Both masculine and feminine ones?"

"Ha, ha, very funny! I see what you're getting at Francois! And I can't say you're wrong here, this place is a synonym for so many encounters and divers and varied adventures... You know I've always been a lady's man."

"Let's just say that you do have quite a reputation, Jacques."

"Really? I had no idea that I was conveying an image like that. But to tell the truth, it's not exactly false. You have to admit that you meet so many people in these international seminars! All sorts of different nationalities: Americans, Japanese, Africans or Italians. Plus, it just takes two minutes to go from the huge amphitheater to your hotel room! Ha, ha! Blame it on the organizers!"

"Sure, it's their fault! Your attraction to women has nothing to do with the way these seminars are organized. You're in charge of your choices."

"Hmm. Choices, talk about a complicated notion. Life is full of choices to be made. Your choice of a career, of women, choices of fate. Each second that goes by is conscious or unconscious choice, whether it's been chosen or forced on you."

"Wow," replied N'Gapet, cutting him off, "you're starting a subject that's much too philosophical for me. I'm throwing in the towel here! Why don't you tell me about your university projects?"

"Well, you know projects are a thing of the past for me now. I'm sure you know that 2005 will be my last year here. I'll be retired in December. I'll be hanging up my gloves, I've had a great life as a doctor, a university career that was fantastic, what else can a guy of my age ask for? Now I'm stepping down; I want to take advantage of the years I've got left to travel, meet up with my friends wherever they are in the world, and you're one of them, Francois!"

"You're certainly welcome to come see us at Lambarene. Weren't you born in Alsace? Like the good Doctor Schweitzer who built our hospital. But come on, you're not an old man yet!"

"Yeah, sure. Seventy-one in three months, that's what I'd call over the hill!"

"You deserve to retire my dear colleague. You gave all your time and knowledge to our science: medicine. You're the global leader in the field of gynecology and genetics. Back home we quote you a lot, believe me."

"You're flattering me, Francois."

Jacques took another sip of his champagne.

"But you're not completely wrong!" he added with a laugh.

Francois N'Gapet joined him in drinking.

"After all these years, what memories do you have of your activity, Jacques?"

"Ah. The sixty-four-thousand-dollar question! What's left of a whole life of hard work? What really impacts a doctor or professor right before he's going to retire? And first of all, is being a doctor a job or a vocation? And which of these is the noblest? Teaching? Research? Or healing? Between a major scientific discovery and saving one life, which of the two has the most value?"

"Or in your case, my dear friend, creating a life."

"It's true, I created, or at least contributed to the creation of a life... or in other words, I helped people who couldn't give birth naturally actually be parents."

"You're a modern-day Doctor Frankenstein!" chuckled Francois N'Gapet, exaggerating his African accent.

"Ha, ha! I just hope I didn't create any Creatures!" Siethbüller replied with a laugh.

Professor N'Gapet joined him.

"Seriously though Jacques, you were a key player in our specialization and your contribution in the field of medically assisted procreation will remain an essential one."

Jacques Siethbüller looked over to the business district in La Défense, towards the *Grande Arche*, a symbol of modern Paris.

"See, Francois, everything is changing around us, timeless Paris is becoming a modern city, medicine is progressing, sciences are changing. What a difference between the eighties and today! Just think about how genetics have contributed to making conception easier. Plus, all the collateral damage that it could incur."

"You're right, Jacques. Sorting embryos to avoid genetic diseases, that's serious progress!"

"Without a doubt, my dear colleague, without a doubt," Professor Siethbüller seemed to be thinking out loud here, looking outside at something, thus remaining silent for a while.

"You're not feeling well?" N'Gapet asked, a bit worried. Jacques suddenly seemed to snap out of his daydreaming.

"I'm fine, perfectly fine. I was just thinking of abuses that are possible: eugenics, or how to choose a pure race, stuff like that. The type of utopia that the Nazis preached and that would be so easy today for any scientists who were brainwashed."

"It's true, you really have to be careful when you manipulate human genes, oocytes, and embryos."

"Right Francois, very careful. And much more so at a global scale than with just a simple individual."

Francois N'Gapet took another sip of champagne.

"You mean, for example, choosing the sex of your child, his skin color, the color of his eyes and hair. Chinese people would only want male children and Neo-Nazis would be capable of creating clones with blond hair and blue eyes."

"All these give rise to ethical and medical questions. Hippocrates hadn't thought of genetics or else he would have included that in his famous Oath!"

Jacques Siethbüller took a deep breath and put a hand on his colleague's shoulder.

"How long have we known each other Francois... thirty years? You're my friend, at least I hope so."

"Of course I am Jacques!"

"My career is nearly over, who knows, maybe my life too."

"Oh come on Jacques," N'Gapet protested.

"Let's just say that I'm nearing the finish line then... Francois?"

"Yes?"

"There's something I'd like to tell you."

Chapter 2

Besançon, February 23, 2015

GUSTS of chilly wind were blowing down the paths of Chaprais Cemetery where a small crowd of people were gathered around a large gaping hole.

At the bottom there were two coffins, side by side.

"We are gathered here together today for a double punishment under the merciful eyes of Our Lord," said the priest with greying temples and a bald head, in a sing-song voice.

On the edge of the tomb, Chloe clutched Leo's hand tightly to show him she was there for him, that she loved him and was determined to support him in the tragic events that happened just a few days ago.

"God works in mysterious ways," the priest

continued. "How can we interpret his intentions in such circumstances? Why did he call back to Him this loving couple, united around their child, you Leo, you who are the symbol of their love? This love which is the greatest thing the Almighty has created."

Leo wasn't paying attention to the priest's words. All they were for him were murmurs and sounds in his head bent down because of the double bereavement he was now affronting.

He could feel the pressure of his sweetheart's fingers though and vaguely looked around at the faces surrounding him, these few friends and family members standing around that awful hole.

He recognized some of his friends: Paul, Marc, Virginie, Vincent, and Sarah. People he'd known when he was a kid, or later on in school, or even colleagues he now was close to.

He also recognized Loic, his father Sacha's best friend, a nice stout man, nearly bald, usually with a peaceful smile.

On the other side of the grave, he thought he recognized Aline and Serge, her husband, proof that opposites did attract. She was a small brunette with blue eyes, and he was a huge giant with a jutting chin and the oft broken nose of a semi-professional boxer. He remembered that Aline was his mother Noemie's best friend and that they worked together as teachers at the same school. Noemie taught French.

"Now let us gather together to pray for Sacha and Noemie's eternal rest. Let us accompany them to the Lord in heaven..."

"Bla, bla, bla," Leo thought when listening to what the priest was saying. It reminded him of advertising he'd often seen on TV for cheese that he liked when he was a kid and he inadvertently smiled.

Leo and Chloe were facing the priest. On both sides of the tomb, they were lost in their thoughts, there where in a few days, when the coffins would be covered by the earth, there would be a new marble tombstone where people would be able to read:

Sacha Terebus – 1955 – 2015

Noemie Kapinsky - 1959 - 2015

He made out other faces. Leo recognized Catherine, his mother's twin sister, so his aunt, though they nearly ever saw each other. She lived in the south of France on the Basque coast and Besancon was *"so terribly far away and so cold, I'm sure you understand,"* as she often repeated in her high voice with a wannabe high-class accent. Plus, Catherine had married well with "Charles the Neurologist," someone who didn't mix with just anyone nor just anything... *"Football, it's so middle-class... golf is played on grass too, but it's much more refined, don't you agree?"*

She had come for her sister's funeral though... But wasn't planning on staying to support her nephew... Winter vacation was coming up fast and she would be spending it in Megeve with Charles, on the slopes... Sure, it was cold there too, but the snow was surely whiter than in Besancon, where the first flakes had begun to fall on the oak coffins.

"Funny what goes through your head at times like this," Leo mused.

"And now, my dear brethren, I'd like to invite you to throw a bit of earth on Sacha and Noemie's grave. Don't forget what was written in the holy Bible, in *Genesis* 3:19: '*By the sweat of your face you shall eat bread, till you return to the ground, for out of it you were taken; for you are dust, and to dust you shall return.*'"

The deacon assisting the priest walked up to Leo with a recipient full of this notorious earth that the priest had blessed. Leo took a bit and looked at it seriously before throwing it into the hole.

It made a sound he'd never heard before, one that he'd never be able to forget.

Father Martin, the priest who had baptized him, threw a few drops of holy water onto the coffins and invited everyone to pay their final respects to the family.

A succession of handshakes, understanding hugs and affectionate kisses on the cheeks.

"My deepest sympathy."
"It's so unfair."
"My deepest sympathy."
"Leo, we're here for you, you know."
"If you need anything..."

"So sorry for your loss."

SOME OF HIS PARENTS' neighbors, whose names he couldn't remember.

His father's boss, who managed some engineering companies in the area.

"What an ordeal... so sudden... such a tragedy..."

Little by little people walked away, some in couples, some with others, some alone.

The snow was falling harder now, covering the coffins with a thin white veil.

Leo handed the priest an envelope.

"Thank you, Father, a moving ceremony," he managed to say between two sobs.

"Be strong my son, the House of our Lord is always open for those who need to talk, stop in and see me."

LEO WAS the last person to leave the cemetery, holding Chloe's arm. Two undertakers were holding their shovels while a third one turned the key on the yellow mini-Caterpillar excavator. Death in the twenty-first century. A gust of wind blew through the alleys of marble slabs.

A bit farther into the cemetery, at the end of a path with cedars on both sides, a silhouette who had remained immobile and discrete during the ceremony walked up to the funeral home employees. Almost like a dark shadow gliding up that the snowflakes somehow seemed to miss.

His arms crossed, a hat down on his head, the silhouette was dressed in black, as were most people who came here, and walked up to the hole that had already been half filled.

The excavator operator stopped working.

"Perhaps you'd like to be alone for a moment? We can come back, there's no emergency you know!"

This person, who had discreetly remained in the background during the ceremony, didn't bother to answer the employee.

After a few minutes of silence and contemplation, he opened his mouth.

"Adieu Sacha… Adieu Noemie."

Finally, the silhouette left as discreetly as it had come, walking towards the exit, leaving the deceased couple, were six feet under, to their eternal rest, united in death as they had been in life.

Chapter 3

Besançon, June 2015

LEO WOKE up next to Chloe who shared his life and this comfortable three-room apartment in Besancon. He had a twinge of sorrow this morning and had decided to do something about it.

"I want to go back there... I want to see..."

He was finally ready to go back to his parents' house, something he couldn't seem to do since that terrible Sunday...

... THAT DAY WAS MUCH MORE than a simple twinge, much more painful than a muted oppression. That afternoon was like a rupture. The news that he'd received by phone had penetrated his ear before spreading like wildfire up to his brain.

At first, he was unable to assimilate the meaning of what the policeman had told him, an ordinary man, though probably quite used to making difficult phone calls like this. Despite his chilly voice, the officer had been able to conserve and impart a bit of humanity, warmth, and compassion in his words.

Leo heard himself respond in a weak voice to Officer Laplace, from the Besancon police station. He remembered hearing his own voice, like a distant echo coming from his entrails. Without even understanding what he was calling about, he had a feeling of foreboding, saying that yes, he was Noemie and Sacha Terebus's son, worrying why the police were suddenly interested in his parents.

When the voice, millions of light years away, on the other end of the line, explained himself, pain - after it had hit his brain and he'd understood it - irradiated all throughout his body like intense burning. The same pain went up and down his backbone, as if welding his vertebrae together into a bar of iron reddened by the flame of a blacksmith torturing him. He stood up straight as a fence pole, his legs paralyzed, sunk into the ground, giving him the impression that they'd been cast into a concrete block. He was gripping the phone so tightly that his joints had turned white, his bones seemed to wrinkle his skin.

Then the pain invaded his bloodstream: Leo

mentally followed its path, feeling it leave his bent fingers, go up his left arm to his shoulder, invade his carotid before going straight to his heart, like an arrow. Unbearable pain, a vice imprisoning his heart, each word the police officer uttered tightened the knob one more notch, squeezing his muscle of life until it nearly burst.

Only tears could free him.

They were still falling when he walked into Officer Laplace's office. He got up, walked to him and with a frank handshake, conveyed all the warmth that he could under the circumstances.

Eyes blurred by tears, Leo listened to the man expressing his sympathy. He thought he'd thanked him before sitting down while the man explained to him that he would have to be brave, that he'd have to officially identify the bodies, which could be very difficult, that the circumstances of the drama - they were talking about an accident, someone who had refused the right-of-way, maybe fallen asleep - had made his parents' faces hard to recognize.

They both walked to the morgue of the neighboring hospital. Nothing on the walls, a chilling silence, sanitized odors meant to camouflage the worst of all smells, that of bodies that had lost all their vital essence.

Leo nearly fainted when the doctor pulled the white sheet down. The vice surrounding his heart jumped another notch. Despite the bruises, the cuts, blisters and burned skin, he had to face the facts: his father and his mother, the two people that were the most important in his short life, the two people who had conceived him, who were at the origin of his presence in this world, were there, cold, lying on the cold grey marble slab.

HE WANTED to go up to the attic to try and find some souvenirs, some traces of the time when he and his parents were still a family. Now, this unit had been torn apart, he was alive, though dying in his head, and his parents whose life had been cut short, stolen from them by a drunk or at least reckless driver who didn't see the STOP sign.

"I'd like to find, I don't know, some pictures, postcards, letters, images of before…"

All these little testimonials, these small impressionist items that prove you're alive, but that all too often, after about twenty years, when you need to make room, people keep so much stuff, don't they - end up in bags or shoeboxes, tin containers, either carefully labeled or just thrown in, reflections of a mishmash life, or on the contrary, a well-organized one.

"I'm afraid to go alone," said Leo with a sob.

"Hey, I've got your back. I'm coming with you," said Chloe, running her fingers through his hair, her head lovingly resting on his chest. "It'll be easier that way, you don't want to do stuff like that alone."

They had a quick cup of coffee in their little kitchen and a few pieces of toast with blackberry jelly, then Leo took his parents' keys that were hanging in the vestibule. Just a double, you never know.

Leo hadn't used his own keys to go to his parents' house for years. For the past three years since he decided to share his life with Chloe, and consequently her apartment, he'd only been back to see them in the evening or maybe Sunday at noon. He had quit saying *at home*, now he said, *at my parents' house*. His room had now become the *spare room*.

Chloe put the parking brake on in her pink Twingo.

"Here we are. Are you going to be okay?" she asked, opening her door.

She'd found a parking place not far from their front door. The white electric gate for the house in the Bregille neighborhood, a chic district in the suburbs of Besancon, was of course locked. Leo didn't have the remote, though he did have the small key letting pedestrians in. His hands were shaking, he had trouble getting it in.

"Give it to me sweetie," Chloe whispered to him, taking it.

The gate creaked slightly as it opened, seemingly occupying all the acoustic space around them. Sounds of the city now seemed far away.

"What am I going to do with this house?" Leo

wondered out loud. "Like it's paid for, I could - we could - even move in, we'd have lots of room.... but I can't imagine that right now."

"I understand. But you know there's no rush, you don't have to decide stuff like that right now. Give it some time."

They went across the lawn using the little path with its Japanese stepping stones and got to the front door. On their left, an empty space reminded Leo that before, there was a Volvo V60 parked there, one that today was just a hunk of crumpled metal, flat tires and broken glass.

"I feel like they're still here, behind the door and they'll open it for us," said Leo.

But when they opened it, there was just a deserted and silent room waiting for them. Of course, for the past four months, nothing had changed, everything had remained as it was before the accident, when they drove to see their friends on that ill-fated Sunday. Noemie's boots were at the foot of the coat rack, one of Sacha's jackets was hanging on it.

Chloe tried not to catch Leo's anxiety.

"I'm going to open the shutters! Let some light in here."

As usual, the house was nice and clean, just like Noemie, always orderly and meticulous.

Walls covered with photos: Noemie and Sacha on their wedding day, Leo as a little kid carrying a ball, Leo ready for school wearing a red artificial leather tie and a checkered sweater that dated him terribly, Leo as a teen wearing a judo kimono, Leo as an adult the day he graduated with his degree as a luxury watch designer, Leo here, Leo there, you could tell his parents loved him.

"You wanted to see some photos? Plenty of them here!" "I know all these by heart!" "You think they've got other ones? Maybe in the office?"

"I just realize now that I've never seen any 'oldies but goodies,' in photo albums, except for the ones hung all over here or on their tables or on the bookshelves. And except for this wedding picture, I don't think I ever saw anything taken before. That's why I think maybe going up to the attic might be a good idea. Actually, I have never gone up there since they bought this house, five years ago. I have no idea what I'll find up there."

They went through the laundry room to go up to the attic.

The light that made its way through the roof with thin beams, the dry heat, the characteristic smell of dust and above all, the view of a symbolic object made Leo segue into his schoolboy's shorts in just a blink...

"Look!" he said as soon as he'd set foot in the attic. "My bike! The one I split my lip on!"

He must have been about ten when he fell off his red bike, a BMX with pieces of cardboard stuck into the spokes to imitate the sound that older kids' scooters made. A bit nostalgic, Leo looked at the front wheel that was bent, the crooked handlebars as well as one of the pedals full of mud that must have been years old.

When you're ten, you're intrepid. A bike, the symbol of freedom allowing you to get away from it all and live adventures that adults had become incapable of sharing.

During one of these outings Leo had his bike accident. Rushing down a dirt path as fast as he could, wind blowing through his hair. The little pieces of cardboard in his spokes filled his ears with an intoxicating buzz. Lost in his imaginary world - this time he was a motorcycle cop in New York - he missed the curve on his left and hit the brakes suddenly: but the wrong one, the front brake! In half a second he was thrown off his bike, sailed over the handlebars and ended up on a side of the rocky path. But Leo walked home without crying, next to his crumpled bike. Proud to prove to his parents that he was now a young man, as this accident had symbolically shifted him from the world of childhood to the world adults lived in, adults who don't cry anymore...

Life is an endless cycle, isn't it? An accident that took him away from his crybaby world, and fifteen years later another accident - this one worse, as he was not directly implicated in it - revived the hidden tears of his childhood, the tears adults think are buried for good, yet they remain, inside, hidden behind a smokescreen of dignity, one that is always ready to overturn the seawall of pride, that adults have with their prudishness.

Chloe saw tears welling up in his eyes.

"It'll be okay honey. You want to keep on looking or should we go downstairs?"

Leo ran his fingers across his old BMX's frame, making a furrow in the dust, like a path leading to the heart of his memories.

That's what he'd come up to the attic to do, to open a path towards the past, the possibility of reliving it, seeing a photo, seeing his parents once again.

"I'll be okay. I really hope I find something here. Time to get down to work," he joked, continuing to rummage around.

They remained in the attic for several long minutes, seeking an eventual family Grail. They lifted up old mite-bitten covers, pushed away several dusty spiderwebs, flipped through several old books, opened boxes full of baby clothes, brown envelopes full of old bills, wondered what these old knick-knacks could have possibly been used for.

His dreams suddenly came true.

"Here we go! Look at this tin box. In movies that's where they often find old souvenirs, right?"

"Open it!"

Leo lifted the dusty cover. The metallic box was covered with dots of rust. Despite the waning light in the attic, he could see lots of photos, postcards, letters and notebooks inside it.

"Ali Baba's cave," he said, lifting up a few photos. "Can't see much here though. It's getting late, we can look at this later on at home."

They went back down, closed the shutters, and left. Leo noticed that the mailbox was overflowing.

"With all that advertising, it's not surprising! The key must be in the front hall."

"Bring back a shopping bag too while you're there. We'll dump everything in it, and we can sort it all out later and keep the important mail."

"I'm going to have all sorts of paperwork to do," complained Leo, just thinking of it.

They took out two armfuls of mail and put it in the bag, making sure they'd closed the door and gate and went into town in their Twingo.

They were holding a tin box and a mountain of papers that they couldn't even imagine what they were hiding, even less so, the importance of it all. Without realizing it, Leo had set himself up for several nights of insomnia.

Chapter 4

Besançon, June 2015

COMFORTABLY SEATED ON THE COUCH, Leo and Chloe were cuddled against each other, both staring at an old school notebook with its yellowish pages, its cover warped by humidity and its pages covered with a refined and slightly slanted handwriting.

"That's my mom's handwriting, no doubt about that."

He'd found a notebook at the bottom of the metallic box he'd taken from his parents' attic, beneath a heap of little knick-knacks, paltry souvenirs, as well as photos, postcards, letters and other emotion-filled personal belongings.

He'd discovered several yellowed and dog-eared photos of him and his parents on the beach in

Vendée, where they usually went on vacation, on a swing, or in his grandparents' house. But also, some photos taken before he was born. Part of his life he'd never even imagined.

"Look at this one," he said happily. "What a nice-looking couple!"

Here, his parents were holding hands, walking down a shady path leading to a lake. He wondered if they'd already talked about having a child then. What was their relationship like in this picture he couldn't really date? Had they known each other for a long time? Had they already thought of living together? During this bucolic walk, had they talked about having children? They seemed so happy here! Hand-in-hand, twinkling eyes, contented grins…

This idealized image of the two lovebirds walking down to the lake had triggered new and irrepressible tears, perhaps tears of joy, like when you watch a movie that has a happy ending.

Under this photo Leo found the notebook he was holding, and when he opened it to the first page, he could read the title his mother had written, a short but ever so promising one: *My Future Child.*

"What the heck?" wondered Leo, flipping through it. "I had no idea that my mom ever wrote anything! It's like a novel."

"No, look," said Chloe, cutting him off, "there are dates, it's more like a diary."

"Oh my god, that's crazy… My mom's diary… I don't know if I should be reading it."

"You know, if she really wanted it to be a secret, she would have destroyed it rather than putting it away in the attic."

"You're right. Anyway, it's too tempting. Listen: *"February 20, 1986. Yesterday, when we were strolling hand-in-hand on the banks of the Doubs, Sacha told me he'd like to have a baby.'*

5

My Future Child

February 20, 1986

YESTERDAY, *when we were strolling hand-in-hand on the banks of the Doubs, Sacha told me he'd like to have a baby.*

I decided to write this all down here in this notebook, this marvelous adventure we'll have as we "create" a child, the joy of starting a "family," this magical word uniting Sacha and myself, the one that only exists when a couple comes together and gives birth to a new being, one that is both the addition or the multiplication of the two original ones, into a new and unique being!

Nine months, maybe a year, starting from tonight when I'll stop taking those birth-control pills I've been on for so many years. One year, like a magical interlude - at least, in our imagination - in a life where happiness is often so difficult. A year that I never want to forget! But as you always forget as time goes by, with this diary, I want to leave a lasting tribute to this human adventure, the one that has fulfilled women from the beginning of time, though each time it is a unique, personal and literally intimate story!

So tonight, to "officially" kick off this "mom and dad operation," we went out to dinner at Peppino's, the Italian restaurant where we used to go when we first fell in love a few years ago, and that we've slightly abandoned for other ones. Peppino hadn't forgotten us though, and neither had we. We wanted to honor him with this emotion filled dinner, enjoying orecchiette alla Genovese accompanied with a bottle of Chianti and a dessert of his famous tiramisu, topped off by a to-die-for cappuccino!

Joy on our plates, joy in our hearts! The meal went by as if in a dream. Holding hands, looking each other in the eyes, talking about our projects for the future, we imagined ourselves buying baby clothes, a stroller, designing the decoration for our future baby's room! Would it be pink or blue? Of course, all that is very premature, but I dare any couple who hasn't dreamed about this to criticize me!

We made love when we came back, stronger than ever maybe, but certainly with more passion than the very first time. Our physical pleasure was enhanced by the hope of giving life. Obviously, chances were slim that I'd become pregnant, as my body was still under the influence of those chemical pills, but who cares! This symbol would bring us luck!

LEO RACED THROUGH THE PAGES, literally dazed by what he was reading. He realized that he was holding the manuscript describing the beginnings of his own existence. The thick notebook was covered in writing up till the last page. There was that much to write about something as commonplace as procreation?

"It's incredible, I'm discovering a whole new world, a whole new part of my 'pre-life,'" Leo told Chloe.

"Well, I'm going to bed, I'll leave you with your book, I'm tired. You can tell me what you found out tomorrow. Don't stay up too late honey, love you."

And she delicately kissed her man and let him enjoy what his mother had written a quarter of a century ago.

MARCH 18, **1986**

MY FIRST AFTER-PILL PERIOD! *It didn't happen this time. But we weren't expecting a miracle. All the hormonal chemical effects after years of taking the pill couldn't fade away that quickly. My body, my ovaries, my ovules, they're still conditioned not to give life! My entrails are on strike, revolting against what is nonetheless mankind's goal: renewing itself generation after generation. For thousands of years, human beings unceasingly reproduced to continue to exist, to remain the leading species on the Earth. Then little by little, Mankind invented methods of controlling its soaring population rates. More and more efficient methods when you consider how far we'd come from coitus interruptus to birth control pills, without forgetting spermicides, IUDs, rubbers whatever they were made from, tubal ligation or oophorectomy! And who was that all targeting? Women! It does take two to tango, right? Men didn't have much to think about in this contraception deal. Rubber or not to rubber, that is the question! But who has to remember to take her pill? Who has to check her ovulation periods? Who has to - in case of an accident - or uncontrollable passion "do what has to be done" making you regret those fleeting minutes of ethereal pleasure? Who?*

But now that's not Sacha and my problem. Quite the opposite. Now it's "full steam ahead towards fecundation!" Long live ovules! The Formula 1 Grand Prix for spermatozoids, the race to the Ovary! More selective than your university SATs, more haphazard than the Lottery, only one winner out of the millions racing towards the Big Egg... With Sacha we have fun comparing the arrival of a spermatozoid to the surface of the ovule to that of Neil Armstrong, a minute human on the huge moon. One small step for the spermatozoid, one giant step for our household!

LEO EASILY RECOGNIZED his mom's style. Always serious, no mistakes, but suddenly able to crack a joke or be witty. This thought, these words, sparked a double feeling of heartache and joy of being alive in him. You could see this strange duality on his face, tears flowing towards the corners of his smile, while he continued to read the notebook full of moments of life that he, of course, had not known.

∼

APRIL 15, **1986**

MY PERIOD CAME AGAIN *this month, or as we say here, "The English have landed!" How I would have liked to be Joan of Arc to expel them from my intimate territory! This is tiring. They won this time. Is it going to come? Or not? That's the question we keep asking ourselves at the theoretical date when my menstrual cycle is over. Here "theoretical" is real! What can be harder than interpreting signs in a woman's body? Can you really feel and analyze the symptoms inside you? Is this little tightness on my left side a sign of ovulation? And is this sharp pain on my right a sign telling me my ovule has pulled out or is it a symptom of appendicitis? And a hard abdominal wall is indicating that the ovule is going from my fallopian tube, or is it merely indigestion? Who knows? I'm already finding it so hard to know what's going on inside my body that I can well imagine how difficult it must be for Sacha who's living all of this from the outside!*

As my ovulation time is so uncertain, how can we know if our lovemaking is at the right time? And when to do it so it's more efficient? How many days before and after the ovulation peak? And to start with, how long does an ovulation last? I've read that it only lasts for ten minutes! Gotta make sure you aim right! Luckily, sperm can survive for four days in the uterus. That's if they're young and vigorous or old and experienced! Sacha wonders if we should make love every day or if it's better to wait to strengthen his gametes and only do it every two or three days. But will we be able to match our ovulation peaks with our excitement peaks? Won't all of these calculations kill our desire, or spontaneity? Will we become procreation machines or remain two human beings that are in love with each other?

Right now, no panic, just patience! And isn't there an old saying that goes 'Patience is the mother of fecundity?' You never heard of it? Tough luck, it's good enough for me!

NOW LEO WAS GETTING tired and he closed the notebook to join Chloe in their bedroom. She was already sound asleep, so he curled up in her back, as he usually did.

Chapter 6

Besançon, June 2015

WHEN CHLOE GOT up the next day, she found Leo already sitting at the counter in their little kitchen, in front of a cup of still steaming coffee. His hair was a mess, his eyes vague.

"Looks like someone just got up," she whispered in his ear, kissing him on his lobe.

He smiled back at her. A strained smile, with worried eyes, nearly a frown.

"Is something wrong?" she asked. "You didn't sleep well? That notebook is bothering you?"

He finally shook out of his daydreaming and showed Chloe a huge kraft envelope.

"You know what this is?" he asked.

"An envelope! So what's my prize?" she joked, trying to make him laugh.

"I don't think there's prize here. But it's really strange."

"Where's it from? And who is it for?"

"That's what's weird. I found it in all the mail that was in my parents' box, mixed in with the advertising flyers."

As if he were trying to prove this, Leo pointed at the various piles of mail on the counter.

"This morning, as I couldn't sleep, I made myself a cup of coffee and looked at that bag with all the mail in it. So I decided to sort it all out, that way it wouldn't take up so much room plus that would be one less thing that needs doing. I said that I'd have to take care of a lot of pain in the ass stuff: bills, official letters, taxes, all that, lots of things I'd have to do like contacting suppliers, creditors, cancel their subscriptions, managing the succession, all that stuff."

"I know honey, you feel like you're all alone to do that. But I'm here you know, I can help."

She tenderly rubbed his neck.

"I know I can count on you, sweetheart. See, I've got three piles here: advertising junk I'm going to toss, bills and official mail. And then this envelope that doesn't fit into any of these three categories."

He handed it to her, she read it, and found herself without words.

Two words on the brown kraft envelope: *For Leo*, handwritten.

"Holy shit! This is crazy!" she finally said. "It's open. What was in it?"

"This is where it gets crazier. Take a look."

He handed her a piece of stationery from the Besancon Mercure Hotel, that had these words written on it:

"Leo, I hesitated to send this to you, but this is what your father wanted, and I have to respect this."

"Holy shit," Chloe repeated.

"You already said that!"

"Sorry, I can't think of anything better."

"Yeah, I had the same reaction."

"It looks like a woman's handwriting, but then I'm no specialist. So what's in it?"

∼

AN HOUR BEFORE, alone in the kitchenette, Leo had hesitated for a long time, contemplating the padded envelope addressed to him. Where could it have come from? Who had put it in the mailbox? And when? It didn't have a stamp on it. Questions he had no answer to as he ripped open the self-adhesive tape closing it.

He carefully took out the piece of paper, unfolded it and looked at the unknown handwriting on it. Just a few words, but heavy, dense ones, simple words that he'd never be able to forget.

"Leo, I hesitated to send this to you, but this is what your father wanted, and I have to respect this."

When he read this sentence, it was like an internal thunderclap. He remembered the day the accident took place.

Nervously, his fingers trembling, he ripped open the sides of the case and grabbed the brilliant circle inside it, immediately dropping it. When he picked it up, he could read these words, words that were stronger than those in the letter:

"To my Son".

∽

CHLOE LOOKED at the laptop that was open and running right here in the kitchen. Then back at the CD.

"Did you look at it?"

"I was afraid to, all alone," replied Leo. "I wanted to wait for you. I've got this feeling that it would be too much for me, all alone. Like, just think of it: an anonymous envelope, that someone visibly put in my deceased parents' mailbox, with a paper inside addressed to me like they know me and talking about my father and then this CD-ROM that my dad seems to have burned for me…"

"You're right, it is scary," Chloe agreed. "We can watch it together if you want."

"You've got enough time?"

"I don't start school till ten today. Hand it over."

Chloe took the CD and put it into the laptop.

LEO, his eyes filled with tears, looked at the computer with his father's frozen face on it. They had watched all of it, listened to everything, assimilated what was being said, both the atmosphere and the details.

The CD-ROM started off with an audio file of a song that Leo had already heard without really paying attention to its sense. So for the very first time he *listened to* rather than just *hearing* this song by Michel Sardou entitled *"Mon Fils"* [My Son] and was touched by its words.

There was also a slideshow with a photo of his parents, when they were young, then the three of them, then one of his dad alone, a closeup, looking right at Leo while Sardou was singing.

"MON FILS, *essaye de me comprendre [Try to understand me, son]*

Je ne sais pas bien m'y prendre [I'm not very good at this]

Et puis c'est pas facile à dire... [And it's not easy to say...]"

SO, what his father was going to tell him must have been so hard for him to say that he had to use someone else's words via this technological artifice.

. . .

"MON FILS, *tu sais dans l'existence [Son, you know in life]*
Il y a des différences [There are differences]
Que désormais tu dois apprendre... [That you now have to learn...]
C'est jamais noir ou blanc [It's never black or white]
Mais d'un gris différent [But different shades of grey]
Comme font les reflets dans la cendre... [Like reflections in ashes...]"

THE SLIDESHOW that Sacha had prepared was so well done that these words seem to come right out of his mouth. Leo was no longer looking at an image on a screen, but he was looking at his father, back from the dead, listening to him.

"MON FILS, *je te parle comme un homme [Son, I'm speaking to you as an adult]*
Parce que tu es un homme [Because you're an adult]
Et que moi j'ai bientôt fini...[And for me life is almost over...]"

THIS *ALMOST* WAS TOO MUCH! This simple word had triggered, through its connotations, new and bitter tears.

. . .

"J'ESSAYE DE *t'expliquer [I'm trying to explain]*
Que tout peut arriver [That anything can happen]
Que rien d'humain n'est éternel [That nothing lasts forever for people]
Même quand les sentiments s'en mêlent... [Even when it concerns feelings.]"

THE SONG STOPPED HERE, with Sacha repeating the words. A voice that came from the unknown:

« SURTOUT QUAND LES *sentiments s'en mêlent ! [Especially when it concerns feelings!"]*

LEO KNEW how gifted his dad was in IT. He remembered seeing him, for hours on end, glued to the family PC, fiddling with files, creating web sites or blogs, mixing songs or compressing DVDs into DIVXs. He taught him loads of things even when he was just a little kid, sitting on his knees, teaching him what to do with the keyboard and mouse, later on how to browse through the internet, giving him all his precious tips.

Leo easily recognized his father's IT dexterity in this multimedia assembly. He couldn't take his eyes off the slide show that summed up all the key points in their family's life, with his father's words in the background.

SON, *my dear Leo, I'd like to speak man to man with you, because what I've got to say to you is much too important for just a casual conversation. I hesitated in this confession, wanting to spill the beans when you were eighteen. I said to myself that then you'd be old enough to understand it. The problem though, was that I wasn't old enough to tell you! Talk about a coward, a father who's afraid to talk to his son...*

Consequently, as I was incapable of talking to you when I was alive, I hope that you'll hear this confession as late as possible, as this will mean that we spent a lot of time together! If you hear it soon, that could only be the consequence of a stupid accident that happened to me.

Whatever though, I'd like you to listen very carefully to this confession, as it will give you the key to unlock the comprehension of your existence. I hope that after this CD is finished, you'll know who you really are.

I think your mother touched on some aspects of our lives when we were younger. I know that she had a notebook that she regularly wrote in during the most intense times of our little family saga. On the other hand though, I don't think she knew anything about this IT confession I'm making here. But who knows! I think that in each couple, in each family, some secrets are quite often open secrets. Each person knows what the other is hiding, but always makes sure for some reason, to let the other know that he knows, and vice-versa! Old sayings often say that a couple that wants to stay together should never hide anything from their spouse, put all their cards faceup on the table, because communication is the key to staying in love. Your mom and I talked a lot, but we both did have our little secret gardens! And that's where I'd like to take you today, my dear son.

But watch out! It's no extraordinary garden, like in Monsieur Trenet's song, I'd even say it's been pretty neglected! It's nothing like a prim and proper English garden, nor a delicately sculpted French one, or even less a patient Japanese garden with its perfect bonsais, refreshing cascades and perfectly trimmed bushes. You'll be discovering thistles, stinging nettles, out-of-control-weeds, broken statues and uprooted trees. Arm yourself with a psychological machete and let me bring you back to the past.

There'll be more than one revelation. So many things to get off my chest. My heart though, has always been, and still is today, for your mother, and of course for you too!

I'd like to tell you about Noemie, your mom.

I'd like you to know how she became my life's revelation; how much I love her and why I love her. She deserves this. Maybe I'll be telling you things I never told her.

You already have a vague idea, but I'd like to start by telling you how we met. You mother and I are living examples of what is called "love at first sight!"

7

Sacha's CD-ROM

We were both students when we met. That was back in 1980. She literally *fell* onto me. The expression *to fall in love* was certainly true in our case. We lived on the same floor, in cheap student housing. Identical studios, very impersonal furniture, but functional stuff, and all of this in a three-story grey and wind and rain battered building. To go upstairs, and we were on the last floor, you had to walk up concrete steps that were halfway exposed outside meaning you got the best of the rain, snow or hail for the same price! One evening, on February nineteenth, about seven at night, it was already dark and slippery. Your mom was coming back, carrying her shopping bags, her book bag and purse, as if she were a mule or a donkey heading up the mountains! And I was running up the steps right after her. And I could add, luckily so, because right at that moment, the person who would become your mother slipped, heading down backwards by the force of dear Newton's gravity.

Fate had united us forever.

Instead of breaking some bones on the slippery steps, she found herself in my arms, looking down at all her shopping scattered all over. We remained like that, stupefied, for a lapse of time that seemed an eternity to us. Her head was looking back, her eyes looking right into mine. Then she blinked and said something I would never in my entire life forget.

"My mom always told me that one day I'd meet my Guardian Angel."

"Oh yeah?"

An intelligent response, wasn't it? I could have answered her with so many things, less commonplace, something that better fit her romantic tirade. But in real life, and you'll realize this as you get older, things are not at all like they are in the movies nor in Harlequin romance novels.

I walked back up to her studio with her after helping her pick up her mungo beans, rice galettes and mushrooms. We started talking together as all students do. *"What are you majoring in?" "Not too stressed out by midterms?" "Are you keeping up with your courses with all this homework?"* Sentences that everyone has either heard or said after graduating from high school! Then, as her studio was tiny, we both sat down facing each other on her single bed. Little by little we had a more constructive dialogue.

As we began to know each other, not as timid, we discovered that we shared a lot of things, from movies by Claude Lelouche up to rhubarb crumble! One thing led to another, and we started talking about when we were little, what we'd done in the twenty years we'd been here on earth. I told her about how I had to have my four premolars pulled out so I could have braces, this horrible greyish device of course efficient in straightening crooked teeth, but one that certainly didn't help me find girlfriends! In return she told me about the tragi-comedy that happened when she was twelve and had her first period at her grandma's place in La Baule...

Swaying between seriousness and hilarity. I dredged out my best jokes, maybe not the funniest ones, but those that I actually remembered the ending to, and she had the delicacy of laughing at them.

"*Make her laugh and you're halfway there*," as the old saying goes... but here I was already lying down on her bed!

Hours flew by like minutes without us even glancing at our watches. No longer timid, we were now peering at each other. We were trying to make out in the pupils of the other that moist glint that never lies, that tiny bolt of lightning symbolizing love at first sight.

As for our hands, it was as if they had a life of their own, touching at 10, meeting each other at midnight, and clutching at three, when our eyelids were getting heavier and heavier.

We were lying next to each other at 5:00 a.m. We didn't have anything else to say so we just fell asleep, innocently, our heads touching and holding hands.

It was only when the alarm went off, surprising us a mere two hours later, that we kissed.

"I've got a course now," she said just after.

Harsh realities of everyday life overtook this time-independent parenthesis of one night.

We both had an espresso, without saying another word, just a smile on both of our lips.

And I went back to my studio, a hundred and fifty feet from hers.

Chapter 8

Besançon, 1986

"AAAH! I can't stand these pimple-faced eighth graders anymore!" complained Aline pushing the door of the teacher's room open. She headed straight to the old, faded beige sofa in the back, where Noemie was correcting her French papers. She continued, sitting down next to her colleague, who was also her best friend.

"Can't even pronounce "*th*" correctly. They just laugh about it and bet on who's going to spit the farthest. They've got their tongues hanging between their teeth, their noses turned up and squinting eyes. 'Ze...ze...ze...se...se...se...' *The, the the*: seriously it's not complicated!"

Aline was inexhaustible on this subject and Noemie finally interrupted her.

"Woah there. Just relax! You're teaching French students, they're not exactly gifted for foreign languages," she said, with this slight Russian accent she'd inherited from her parents.

Born in Odessa, in Crimea, she'd come to France when she was only six, with her father, the famous violinist, Grigor Kapinsky, who taught at the *Paris Conservatoire* for about fifteen years. Then her parents went back to Russia, leaving Noemie and Catherine, her twin sister, to continue their studies in the capital. Noemie spoke fluent Russian, French and English. She also knew basic Spanish so she could legitimately criticize all the deficiencies that French students had in learning foreign languages as well as the way they were taught in the country she had now adopted.

"Why didn't I decide to teach German," continued Aline, still grumbling. "I wouldn't be covered with drops of saliva all day long!"

"Maybe not, but you'd probably have a sore throat with all those guttural "*r*'s" and "*ch*'s. Russian is the most beautiful language! Strong yet flexible, just like me," Noemie said with a laugh.

"Oh! Say something to me in Russian, I love it when you speak that language."

"What do you want me to say?"

"I don't know, whatever you want, what sounds nice, to make me dream or travel through the steppes, anything so I'll forget those pimple-covered faces!"

"*Моё сердце сгорает от любви.*"

"What does that mean?"

"My heart is burning with love."

"Oh! How nice. That's why I love you, Noe! Just a couple of words and I'm smiling again. So is your heart burning for love for me? Or for your little Sacha? You're glowing, what did your good-looking guy do?"

Noemie blushed and smiled even more thinking of her sweetie.

"You can tell?" she asked innocently. "We had a great weekend. Plus I've got something to tell you…"

"He proposed!" said Aline, cutting her off. "Oh! That's awesome! When's the wedding? I'm invited I hope. And who's going to be your maid of honor? Hope you think of me. Who's your best friend? Huh, who?"

Noemie burst out laughing.

"Shhh! Shut up, old Rene's looking at us."

Rene, the old Latin teacher, as dead as the language he kept on trying to teach to his students who couldn't care less about him or his *rosa, rosis, rosam*. He was concentrating on an antique version of Seneca and frowned disapprovingly when he looked at his feminine colleagues.

"Oh! Sorry, Rene. We were just leaving. Hope you like the book! And say hi to Seneca from us!" Aline joked, dragging her friend outside.

"*Juventus stultorum magister*"[1], replied the old Latin teacher.

"*Alea jacta est*"[2], retorted Aline when she walked by.

Both ladies laughed.

As soon as they'd left, Aline continued.

"You already chose a date then? Where's it going to be? Here? Or in Russia?"

"Stop!" Noemie nearly shouted. You're barking up the wrong tree. We're not getting married, that's not a priority."

"So what's the news then?"

"We decided to start a family!"

"Awesome!" replied Aline, hugging her friend. "I'm so happy for you. You know I love kids. Babies are just so cute. So when's it for? You'll think of me when you're choosing a godmother, right? I'm ready."

"You are completely off your rocker. Don't you ever stop talking? A real chatterbag!"

"No, the right word is a chatterbox, Miss Noemiskaia!"

"Whoopsie. "I got it mixed up with 'in the bag.'"

"Anyway, when's the big date then?"

"Come on, we've barely begun. I went off my birth control pills just two months ago."

They went past the guardian's office, waving at him through the window, and went outside. It was recess, and bunches of teens were wandering around. Aline lit up a cigarette.

"So that means that next year you'll be leaving poor little Aline high and dry? What am I going to do without you, all alone with my sputterers?"

"Go buy yourself an umbrella that you can attach to your forehead," Noemie joked.

"How long have you and Sacha been together?"

"Easy. We met at the university in 1980. Six years then."

"That's quite a while! You guys aren't in any hurry! Six years before decided to start a family"

The end of her Gitane cigarette glowed. Aline inhaled the smoke before slowly blowing it out, looking up at the clouds, her eyes half-open. She continued:

"With Serge, we started our family with Celine after having lived together for two years, actually right after we got married."

"Normal. You're always in a hurry! You do everything quickly: you speak quickly, eat quickly, get married quickly, have kids quickly, do you fuck quickly too?"

Aline nearly suffocated with her cigarette smoke.

"Ha! You language nerd: sometimes your vocabulary surprises me! But if you really want to know, Serge often... does it quickly! As for me, I'd like it to be a little bit longer! You know Serge does step on it: when he was a boxer, he didn't want to spend an eternity in the ring. Bing, bang, a right over here, an uppercut there, a left hook, and KO! Pay day, *adios amigos!*"

While she was saying this Aline air-boxed, imitating her husband, indifferent to the amazed looks on the faces of the kids outside.

"Slow down Linette! You're going to knock me out there!" said Noemie, pushing away the little fists of her friend. "He was a good boxer then?"

"Not bad, not bad at all. He won several fights, knocking out his opponents. Though he did lose some the same way. You know, he was a semi-professional. But he wanted to stop when Camille was born. He didn't want to become a vegetable-dad."

"What the heck is a vegetable-dad?"

"It just means that when you're a boxer, you get hit in the head quite often and it's not good for your neurons, especially when you pass out. It doesn't look like much, just a few seconds, but they say that the neurological consequences are enormous. So he hung up his gloves and opened his garage. He still works with gloves on, but now it's so he won't get grease stains on his hands!"

"I get it, not as glorious but more responsible. Like a good dad!"

"Yup! His employees call him Serge Balboa, in reference to Rocky, or else Rocky the Monkey Wrench. He always has a laugh about that. Sometimes he gives them a friendly tap on the shoulder, not full force, of course."

Aline took one last puff from her Gitane and put it out, stepping on it.

"Would he be a good father then?"

"I think so. He's really gentle and at ease with kids. I can tell when I see him playing with my sister's kids, even though we don't see each other very often. Plus I know that he really wants a family, with two or three kids. Especially because he was an only child."

"That's right."

"And I think he really wants to play his role as a father and see me in mine as a mother. I know that he lost his parents too early."

"Really? What happened?"

"I actually couldn't tell you, he never wanted to talk about it. He just said that their last days were painful and that it was a tragic end. And I know it's hard for him to think back on these souvenirs, so I never really insisted."

"That's understandable. Anyway, what a fantastic project you have! And if you need any advice, you can come to see me, I've got plenty of experience. You'll see, when you're pregnant it's magical: for me both times were different, but a tummy that gets bigger and bigger is like magic," said Aline enthusiastically, thinking back. "I'd do it again, no questions asked. But now I'm well over thirty, so it's your turn!"

Right then the bell rang. The colleagues went back into their classrooms. Just before they separated, Noemie made fun of Aline.

"Miss, do you say '*ze, zis, zat*, or *zoze*?'"

Aline pretended she was strangling her with both hands while Noemie opened an imaginary umbrella above her head.

Chapter 9

Besançon, 1986

SACHA SLID a cassette into the hi-fi beneath the television: a collection of slows, from the 60s up till now, 1986. He'd recorded the best of the Platters, Elton John, Telephone, Lionel Richie, without forgetting Whitney Houston. Music began with Still Loving You by the Scorpions and Sacha went back into the kitchen where he'd already uncorked a bottle of Saint-Émilion 1980, the year when they met each other. He picked up the decanter and poured the wine into two glasses, filling them with a magnificent carmine red that looked promising.

He could hear Noemie singing along to Still Loving You in the bathroom, at the end of
He heard the shower: a powerful stream

on her long brown hair; drops rolling down her neck, caressing her tiny breasts, tickling her flat stomach; drops that were still hot that must have found their way between her legs, before running down them and swallowed up by the shower plug. At least that's what happened in Sacha's head who could never resist thinking of his Noemie nude, whatever the circumstances could be. But he perhaps was not an isolated case: don't all men think like this? Those in love, I mean. Or old perverts, who knows?

Now Sacha only wanted one thing: to join her in the shower, at least wash her. Anoint her body from head to foot with her perfumed shower gel and feel her shiver beneath the movement of his palms. But he'd already donned his flannel shirt and his slacks and was busy setting a nice table for them.

He regretfully forced himself to continue and take some candles out from the kitchen drawer. He found two nice pewter candle holders and put two long red twisted candles in them.

He skillfully threw a white tablecloth on the round coffee table in their living room and placed the two candles on it.

In the meanwhile, she'd finished her shower and the Platters had replaced the Scorpions.

ONLY YOU AND *you alone*
   Can thrill me like you do

*And fill my heart with love for only you
Oh oh oh only you…*

A BIT KITSCH, but it always got the job done. Sacha was literally vibrating and started humming when he set the table.

In the bathroom, the hair dryer blowing told him that his wife would soon be out with her beautiful wild and curly hair. He was so looking forward to breathing in the fresh fragrance of her coconut milk shampoo in her hair.

Sacha turned on the oven and slid a pan of appetizers in. Then he started peeling some of the two-dozen jumbo shrimp for the main dish.

This was when Noemie walked in. She was so beautiful she took his breath away. She was wearing her long red dress with a slit in the back: the point of the V began just below her hips, unveiling the curves of this brunette whose hair flowed down.

They'd known each other for six years now and Sacha still couldn't believe his good luck. He loved everything about her, whether she was wearing sports clothes, an evening dress, or nothing at all. He often said to himself that he was really lucky to be loved by a woman who was both beautiful and intelligent.

"More beautiful than yesterday and less than tomorrow," he whispered to her.

Noemie put her arms around him.

"What a Casanova! Too bad your fingers are full of shrimp juice, otherwise you would have been able to touch!" she taunted him.

"You're killing me," Sacha replied. "You just wait!"

"But anyway you're really sexy in your chef's apron! Can I try one?" she asked, pointing at the shrimp he had just peeled.

Sacha slid it between her teeth. Leaving half of it out of her mouth, she slowly brought her lips to Sacha's to share it with him. He bit his half off, then just like The Lady and the Tramp with their spaghetti, they both nibbled away delicately and finished with a deep and salty kiss.

"Delicious," she said. "I'm hungry..."

"For me?"

"First let's eat, then after... who knows?"

While preparing the spaghetti with its citrus and shrimp sauce, they both sipped their Saint-Emilion, in between kisses. They enjoyed appetizers while the pasta was cooking.

After the Platters, they put on Phil Collins, Barbara Streisand, and Diane Tell. After two glasses of Bordeaux and when the pasta was done, Herbert Léonard filled the house with testosterone.

POUR LE PLAISIR: *[Just for pleasure]*
S'offrir ce qui n'a pas de prix, [Give us a priceless gift]

Un peu de rêve à notre vie, [A few dreams in our life]
Et faire plaisir, [And please each other]
Pour le Plaisir… [Just for Pleasure...]

THOUGH THE WATER was no longer boiling, the temperature of the room and the blood pressure of the two lovebirds kept on rising.

Dinner, piping hot, was served: delicious scents of shallots, orange and flat leaf parsley tempted their taste buds.

They sat down at the coffee table, on flat pillows, with only candlelight.

"I'm so happy, darling," said Noemie, looking right into Sacha's eyes. "And we'll soon have a baby here at home."

"I'm happy too."

"And will you still love me, even when I'll be too fat to wear this dress?"

"You will be the most beautiful mother-to-be in the world! But the first thing we have to do is make this baby..."

And, turning talk into action, Sacha leaned into Noemie, nibbling on her mouth, caressing one of her breasts through her dress, pulling one of its straps down.

The young lady, subjugated by Sacha, laid down on the thick carpet, welcoming his weight on her.

When they got back up, a few minutes later, the

spaghetti and shrimp were cold, the candles had burned down and Stevie Wonder was on the phone.

I JUST CALLED *to say I love you*
I just called to say how much I care
I just called to say I love you
And I mean it from the bottom of my heart.

10

Noemie's diary

You know it's crazy, once you start trying, the whole world is different! Wherever I go, to work, to the movies, shopping, in public transportation, waiting at the check-out, wherever I am all I see is pregnant ladies... Big tummies, several months gone, ready to pop. How many maternity dresses, so easy to spot, dresses that I am only dreaming of wearing? Sacha is obsessed with this too, victim of never-ending visions of women with glowing faces each time they touch their rounded stomachs...

I can admit it, because I don't want to hide any of my emotions in this diary: I think we're becoming jealous, envying these couples who "got pregnant" so quickly!

That's the case for some of our friends. We envy them but are certainly not jealous. We're just happy that they're happy. But we also wish that I'd soon be in the same case! It worked for Aline and Serge on the first month! On the contrary, Bernard and Emmanuelle have been trying for over two years now. I'm sad for them, they're so very nice and life hasn't been easy for them.

Okay, the average between the time when you go off the pill and when you get pregnant is eight months (at least that's what my gynecologist told me), so we should be reassured because we've only been trying for four months now. How many months will it take before we stop believing? How long will it take before the jubilation of getting pregnant transforms itself into apprehension when you get your period? And what can I even say about months when my cycle isn't regular... Where we hope for a couple of days, where we're thinking of going into a drug store to buy a pregnancy test that we finally don't even need as I get my period the very next day, as if it were making fun of me?

Sacha and I are starting to toss and turn at night more and more, finding it increasingly difficult to fall asleep.

∼

LEO PUT the cup of herbal tea back down, without actually having enjoyed it, still thinking of what he'd just read.

A few minutes before he had put his mom's diary down, still open, pages against the table, protected by the cover just like a veil masking Noemie's doubt.

While pouring the simmering water over his lemon-lime blossom tea, his thoughts had begun to drift. He'd realized that before reading what his mother had written, he'd never considered pregnancy like this. Everything that he had read up till now on the subject of pregnancy, wanting to start a family, or fecundation, just showed happy families, confidence and success. Everything always happened too quickly, the first time, without the least effort or doubt. But did people want to read books, listen to songs or watch movies that would darken their own dreams? Books too close to daily triviality wouldn't interest anyone. After all, in all the books his mom had read to him when he was little before turning off the lamp, they *all lived happily ever after... all of them, meaning the husband, wife and kids*. Such a typical Catholic sentence, such an idealistic world...

Leo smiled at the gap between fiction for kids and the harsh reality that his parents had undergone to conceive him. He even thought about this improbable song by Fernand Sardou *"Aujourd'hui peut-être"* [Maybe Today], where the orator from Marseille in the south of France had three children only two months after he got married to Therese!

He was still smiling when he picked the book back up.

END OF AUGUST **1986**

For the past couple of weeks both Sacha and I have been finding it hard to have sex. We're completely obsessed by the idea of having "efficient" sex, that we forget to make love, just because we love each other!

Each month, we get stressed as the time for my ovulation comes nearer. We decided to do it just every other day, as we now had to match the length of my ovulation, an optimal renewal as well as the lifespan that sperm have! This rhythm seems the best one to have the best chance of success. Some of my girlfriends say we should do it every day, but my gynecologist agrees with me here.

But we now feel like we are procreation machines, mathematicians of lovemaking, pros in procreation, technicians of controlled sex... and simple pleasure is a thing of the past. We try to believe that this is a mere interlude in our lives, and that once we'll have started a family, our sex lives will be pleasurable and fulfilled, relationships between lovers without any hidden agendas of procreation.

All these ovulatory calculations, copulatory calculations inhibit us, rather than motivating us.

Far from finding pleasure in the act, we have mechanical sex, my body finds it hard to lubricate, Sacha's intimate flag sometimes flies at half-mast, in a sky without any wind! When this happens, he sits up and puts his head between his hands, nearly crying, unable to say a word when his virility doesn't respond. So I try to reassure him without convincing myself that it's not a big deal, that maybe it's not even the right day, that tomorrow or the day after, things will be looking up, or maybe even next month. Bullshit! We have no idea!

Such lucky couples who never had to cross the abyss in

their lives between "Honey, let's make love, now!" and "We have to do it tonight, it's Wednesday! And make sure you don't take a hot bath, you know your gynecologist said it's not good for the sperm!"

Chapter 11

Besançon, June 2015

LEO SUDDENLY WANTED to close the book when he read those last sentences. Too intimate. He wasn't comfortable reading such personal details of his own parents' lives. He had just unveiled a whole part of their lives he'd never even thought of and felt he shouldn't have known. Just like all kids, he'd only thought of his parents as "parents." How could he imagine them making love? Impossible for a child! An intellectual taboo or mere self-deception? Later on, as a teen, when he saw people making love on the TV, had he imagined his parents doing the same thing? He didn't think so, it was something he couldn't fathom.

But there, for the very first time, reading his mom's revelations, he was faced with the brutal reality. His parents had sex! In just one second, it was like he had become a little too curious kid, his eye glued to the keyhole, behind the closed door of his parents' bedroom. He felt like he'd violated their intimacy, *post-mortem* which was even worse. A sexual taboo, on top of the taboo of death...

These thoughts were making him sick, and he needed a breath of fresh air, to distance himself, both physically and mentally, from this book with its burning and unholy secrets.

He went outside. Hands in his pockets, the collar of his jacket raised as high as possible to protect him from that frosty black wind, so well known in this part of France, he walked mechanically. Though he'd left the notebook behind, he couldn't get it out of his mind. Leo imagined his parents' bodies touching each other, caressing each other and coming together as one and that bothered him. Little by little though, this feeling left him and he began to smile. Of course, what had he been thinking? That he'd just popped out of the blue? Or like Gargantua, that he was born through his mother's ear? Or like Eve, from one of Adam's ribs? Or even like Christ, an Immaculate Conception? You can get kids to believe junk like this, stuff like boys are born in a field of cabbages and girls in a field of roses, and then delivered to their parents by a caring stork, but as an adult how is it impossible for you to admit that you'd been the fruit of sexual intercourse between your mother Noemie and your father Sacha...

There's always a tacit taboo on the subject of sex when you're talking about your friends or family. It's pretty rare to hear questions like *"How are things in the bedroom for you two?"* or *"How often are you doing it to optimize your chances?"* or *"Do you both have orgasms?"* when you're having a beer with your friends.

Nonetheless, such hypocritical and innuendos-filled sentences we continue to sputter out. *"We've been trying to start a family for a couple of months now."* Behind this politically correct formulation, that even grannies smile at, if you think of it, this actually means: *"For weeks we've been fucking every other day to try to have a kid!"*

That might shock people, but it does well describe our situation. Two ways of explaining things designate the same act of intercourse and the same creative outcome.

That's how Leo mentally got back on track. Yes, his parents must have "slept together" to conceive him! And if they had fun doing it, well good for them!

And without actually realizing it, he turned around and went back to the apartment where he hunkered down in his armchair before picking up his mother's diary once again.

Noemie's diary

Christmas 1986

I LOVE MY GYNECOLOGIST!

Dr. Lepic is so terribly human, so warm that I can even overcome the never-ending apprehension of the speculum with her nearly maternal gestures. It's like I was a little kid again. When she speaks, the words and the sophisticated music they compose make me feel like I've rubbed a soothing cream over my skin.

I must admit though that I needed something after all these stressful weeks that Sacha and I have gone through. These weeks that go by, without anything happening.

Well, no, not really. A mini alert that made me make an appointment with Dr. Lepic: over a week late... but a negative pregnancy test.

What is going on in my womb? I'd like to be able to spy on the inside to understand how this fabulous feminine anatomy actually works! Had I known, I would have become a doctor like my dad wanted me too and I would have specialized in gynecology! Haha!

So anyway, after this appointment I was serene, not quite so up tight and I hoped once again.

"Ten months," Dr. Lepic said reassuringly, "that's no big deal. I'm sure that if you and your husband just calm down and relax, you'll soon get some good news. Just try for another three months, take a nice vacation, relax both of you, and after you get back, if there's still nothing new, come back and see me. But I'm sure that you won't have to pick up the phone... unless it's to give me some good news."

Chapter 13

Besançon, February, 1987

NOEMIE AND SACHA were standing in line at the supermarket in Chateaufarine. They'd met there after work to do their shopping together. For the past couple of months, they'd multiplied activities together, so that they wouldn't be alone, drowning in their own thoughts. They'd been trying to get pregnant for a year now. What had begun as a source of joy had now become a daily apprehension: why wasn't it working? Why did it work for others and not them?

The romantic evenings they'd spent together seemed like centuries away.

Of course, faced with their failure to conceive, they remained a close-knit couple, but as the months went by with their series of sterile cycles, pressure was growing.

Sacha could only observe Noemie's frustration, her bitterness, her jealousy of other couples for whom it worked.

And that day, at the supermarket, it was the proverbial straw that broke the camel's back. This straw materialized itself as a woman who seemed to be at least eighteen months pregnant and who politely spoke to Noemie, with one hand on her enormous bump and the other holding her groceries.

"Excuse me. Could I cut in front of you? I don't have much and I'm really exhausted."

Sacha quickly turned around when he heard her. He'd seen both the lady's enormous baby bump and Noemie's furious look, as if she was ready to tear her apart. He'd feared what she might say, but she quickly smiled at her.

"Of course. No problem. We're not in a hurry, are we darling?"

Sacha noted her irony but nodded.

"No. Not at all."

"Thank you so very much," the young lady said. "I'm almost due, plus they're twins!"

Noemie would have liked to tell her that she couldn't care less about these indecent details, but she forced herself to smile back at her politely.

She checked out her items, put them back in her

bag and then when she was walking out, thanked Sacha and Noemie one more time.

A few minutes later, when they were driving back, Noemie was still silent and scowling. He'd been trying to joke or just talk about any old thing, but she still refused to answer.

"Come on honey, what's up?"

Noemie kept her eyes on the road, straight ahead, still frowning. Then she suddenly began to talk, like a seawall breaking down because of the waves.

"I'm sick and tired of this! I can't stand all these broads strutting their huge stomachs! And I can't stand the fact that mine is still flat, flat and desperately empty!!! Get it? Sick and tired of this shit!"

"I understand hun," he answered, putting his right hand on Noemie's. "It's hard for me too, but we can't be jealous of them."

"But how can you be so zen? Like you didn't care about having a kid!"

Sacha slowed down imperceptibly.

"Not at all, why did you say that? I want a child just as much as you do. But it's true, maybe it's not as hard for me. We have to be patient."

"Be patient? We've been patient for a year now! And now I'm tired of all this! I don't believe it anymore and I'm sure that if I don't think it'll happen, it won't," she said, pointing at her stomach.

"That doesn't mean a thing," Sacha said, trying to calm her down.

Noemie sighed noisily and looked out the window on her side. She seemed to be thinking something over. She finally decided to get it out.

"Listen honey. I think I need help."

"You don't think I help you enough? I've got your back, you know. We're both in this together."

"You didn't understand me here... I think I need... I think I need more professional and... external help. I'm thinking of consulting a psychologist."

When he heard that word, Sacha turned white as a sheet.

"What do you think about that?" she insisted.

Now it was his turn to remain silent, his hands gripping the steering wheel, his eyes looking at the horizon.

"We could go together if you want. Like it's a problem for both of us, and we're in it together like you said!"

Sacha slammed on the brakes. Noemie nearly hit her head on the dashboard.

"Are you crazy? What the hell's going on?"

He violently turned the steering wheel to the right and pulled over to the side of the road.

"No way," he muttered.

"But why? I'm sure that something like this would be beneficial."

"Beneficial? Bullshit! Psychiatrists, that's a bunch of hogwash! They earn their money from weak people; all they do is stir up shit."

"What are you talking about? Is something wrong? If you don't want to go, fine, but I think I need to. Aline recommended someone to me."

Sacha held his head between his hands with both fists clenched, as if he was trying to soothe a sudden migraine.

"You will not go and consult a quack!" he shouted.

"You're scaring me here..." and Noemie began to cry silently.

"I couldn't care less! It's a bunch of bullshit!"

"Listen, I'm just telling you that I need help and you get all bothered and start yelling, like you're crazy."

Sacha was boiling inside. Trembling.

"Listen, Noe. I want you to understand why I'm reacting like this. I personally don't have a problem with them, but it's linked to my parents."

Noemie paid attention to him, intrigued. She blew her nose noisily. She could see that he was going to tell her something she'd never known.

Sacha continued his story, speaking in monotone, nearly absent.

"I already told you about my parents, didn't I?"

"Of course, but I know that there are things concerning them that you've never told me."

He took a deep breath.

"It's true, you never met them. My mother died in 1977 and my father passed away not even a year after. He'd been diagnosed with prostate cancer about ten years before. He lived with it, it really didn't bother him, though I could see he often was tired. That impacted my mom's moods, she was always much more fragile. She was really sensitive, empathic and took good care of her husband, just like wives did back in the day. Then year after year you could almost see her fading away, and no one could do a thing about it. She tried to hide her unhappiness from us, but she was depressed. She began to consult a psychologist. At that time this was quite rare, and people didn't talk about it. So, she sort of hid this. Sometimes she was really despondent: she could spend days on end without going outside, and sometimes didn't even get up in the morning. She could swing from despondency to euphoria for no apparent reason. Now she would have been diagnosed as having a bipolar disorder. A good day, then a bad one. And no one understood why. She became dependent on her shrink. Going to see him more and more often. And then suddenly, one day, she quit. No one ever knew why at home. Two months later, she hung herself."

"Good Lord, honey... You never told me that, I had no idea."

"It became a taboo subject for my dad and me. After that, he was the one who started wasting away. They were an intensely close couple. His prostate cancer spread, and in less than a year, he was gone too."

Noemie caressed Sacha's cheek tenderly while he continued.

"My dad cried every day for the last couple of months. I heard him curse that psychiatrist, that charlatan who in his opinion, made my mom so much worse instead of curing her. He held him responsible for her death. And if my mother hadn't died so early, so young, my father wouldn't have followed her so closely. So when I hear you talk about all these so-called specialists, you can understand that it frightens me!"

"I understand. But it's not because that's what happened to your parents that the same thing will happen to us!"

Sacha dried his tears. He'd stopped trembling when he finished confiding his secrets. He turned the key and put the car in first gear.

"Honey, please, I'm begging you, don't talk to me anymore about shrinks."

They went back home without another word, both lost in their dark thoughts.

Chapter 14

Besançon, March, 1987

"EIGHT TO EIGHT"! exclaimed Loic. "You want to go to nine or ten?"

"Nine!" replied Sacha while preparing to receive his best friend's service.

He was waiting to see what side Loic would choose and went to the opposite side of the squash court that they rented for an hour per week when they were both available. Loic usually was. He was a chef in his own restaurant, lived alone and needed this weekly hour of squash to try to lose some of his excess weight that he immediately gained back when he tasted all his rich sauce dishes.

Loic hit the little black ball towards the front wall. It powerfully bounced towards Sacha who didn't give it enough time to touch the ground and he volleyed it directly back to the left wall. Then it touched the front wall again, near the window in the angle. And hit the ground before Loic could play it again.

"Nine - eight!" Sacha shouted. "Gotcha this time!"

"Good game," Loic said, shaking his hand.

Both were covered in perspiration after this set of five rounds.

"This does me a lot of good," Sacha said as they walked to the showers.

"You up for next week? Same time, same place, same champion?'

"UM, I don't know if I can make it."

"What's up Sacha? Today you won because you're physically in better shape than me, no doubt about it," Loic admitted, patting his ample stomach. "But it was like you weren't always there on the court. I mean, like you were thinking of something else. Wanna talk about it?"

They took off their clothing and continued their discussion choosing two adjacent showers: that way they could continue to talk while showering. They were the only ones in there.

"Yeah, right now things are pretty tense at home with Noe. It's starting to get long, this baby that we can't seem to have, like we've been trying for over a year now. And it's really hard for her."

"That's normal," Loic agreed. "Maternity, for women, yeah, like it's something that's visceral. They feel that stuff deep down, much more than we do."

"We're going crazy. Like we can't stop thinking about it. That's all we live for and all we dream of. We're obsessed, negatively so."

"Chill! Take a vacation!" Sacha rinsed his hair and grabbed his towel.

"Yeah, we thought about it. But right now, I've got a business trip for a week. I think that maybe it would do us good to take a little break, you know, to have a few days off rather than thinking about this together all the time."

"Where you going?"

"Milan. I'm replacing one of my colleagues on short notice because he's on sick leave and we're negotiating a huge contract."

"Cool! You speak macaroni?"

"Not a word Chef! We'll make do in English or in French."

They got dressed and left the squash clubhouse. Loic waved at him in the parking lot.

"Say hi to the veal cutlets from me!"

"What?"

"The Milanese ones!"

"Ain't you the comedian, Lolo," chuckled Sacha, shaking his hand. "See ya, and glad you lost!"

"I'll make it up to you next time!"

Chapter 15

Milan, February, 2015

THE DRIVER SLAMMED the back doors of his truck, made sure they were correctly attached, and then walked up to the cab, blowing on his cold hands before waving one last time to the cargo handler.

"*Sta per nevicare!*" he shouted back. "*Stai attento Pippo!* "

Ciao, Giuseppe."

Pippo, an overweight Transalpine driver with long hair attached in a greying ponytail, climbed into the cab of his thirty-eight-ton semi. At his age, with his aching knee, he was finding it harder and harder to get behind the wheel. He didn't have the choice though, as he'd always driven semis. Everyone has to make a living, right? So, driving trucks or something else! Well, had he been able to do something else… but that's life, good and bad surprises.

Sometimes he wondered if he'd simply failed. Hours and hours behind the wheel, at fifty-five miles per hour, seeing nothing else but the back of another semi, miles that went by slowly, on sad European highways, stuff that makes people lose all hope. Hours of thinking, thinking about what could have been, if… or if not…

Pippo glanced one more time at his bag he'd thrown into the bunk in his cab behind the seats. His little place. That's where he spent most of his time, more than at home in the outskirts of Milan. His truck had become his home for nearly thirty years now, outside of the ten years that he'd spent in a room not much larger than the bunk, but one that was much darker…

Thirty years he'd been driving from England to Greece, from Spain to Lithuania. Thirty years of sleeping in bunks in semis, taking showers in filling stations on the highway, heating up meals on the hotplate plugged directly into the battery, watching movies all night on the little TV on his dashboard, with the curtains closed in front and on the side windows. A miniature home, actually.

Without forgetting the purring of the other vehicles when they parked next to you, the noisy decompression of the pneumatic brakes, the humming of cars as they whizzed down the three-lane highway not far.

A truck driver's life.

He turned the key, took the parking brake off and carefully accelerated towards the gate of the Pirelli facility. He was hauling a heavy load of new winter tires for this famous Italian brand, the world's fifth largest, also known for its automobile competitions.

He'd hauled tons and tons of tires for them!

This time the payload was for France. He'd need four or five days for the round trip.

He put his right blinker on, drove up to the well-named *Viale Pietro e Alberto Pirelli*, honked three times to say goodbye to the facility's security guard and was off. The beginning of a long trip.

Pippo mentally reviewed his itinerary. He'd memorized dozens of possible routes, which varied according to the seasons, weather, and school vacations. He was still hesitating on which one to take. In February, there was lots of snow in the Alps, it was freezing and that could have an impact. He had two options. Either go north, through Lugano, between Como and Locarno Lakes, then to Switzerland through Andermatt, Luzern and Basel. He'd be taking the Saint-Gothard tunnel then, as the peak was already closed. Or he could go west, through Val d'Aosta heading towards Geneva and then take the Mont-Blanc tunnel.

Whichever one he chose, he'd have to wait for

hours to go through one of these road tunnels, which since the horrible accidents that took place in 1999 in the Mont Blanc tunnel and in 2001 in Saint-Gothard, had become a real headache for professional truck drivers.

Anyway, he'd planned on a small detour after unloading. He had to comply with driving and rest times, that was the law and that was his right. Once he'd unloaded, he'd have a bit of time and freedom to do what he had to do... a little personal detour. This opportunity was too good not to take advantage of it. He'd been waiting for years now. And now because of sheer luck, he had one.

He turned towards the Lake Region. He'd come back through Val d'Aosta.

After his little detour... After...

16

Sacha's CD-ROM

There you go son; you know the beginnings of your own life. That night should have been the departure of a great family life, ending with the arrival of a superb baby named Leo, strong like Leo the lion!

So, you see, it was love at first sight for both of us. Right away we knew we couldn't live without each other, without actually putting this into words. We were in love, that was it. And if love at first sight isn't shared, it's more like a type of fantasy or pathological lie, don't you think? Anyway, we quickly started seeing each other in one of our studios. They were exactly the same! Working on our mid-term exams, side by side, on a bed, tons of paper spread out on the covers. That lasted for three months until we realized that paying rent on two studios was ridiculous, as we only used one. So after my final exams in June, I checked out of mine and moved my stuff a couple doors down. It was a little small for two, but we couldn't have cared less! We kept each other warm and that was the most important thing.

Seems idyllic, doesn't it? Fate had thrown us together - Cupid, the Alchemist - making two lives into one. Love then moved in with us. Two turtle-doves, living on love, water and bread! This saying was almost true, but instead of water and bread we enjoyed good restaurants and great wine! Just as romantic! We often went to Peppino's, this Italian place with its homemade *tiramisus*. And then a few years later, we went to the same restaurant to celebrate our decision to start a family and that's when your mom started writing in her little diary. She often went into the office to pen some secrets, after we'd finished eating. Of course, I never snooped, I never tried to read what she'd written, that was for her, I think it helped her during those long months where all we focused on was trying to have you.

I'll get back to that later because I've got stuff to tell you too about this, stuff she never even imagined. But before that, I'd like to tell you more about these wonderful years, these six years that went by between when we first met and when your mom and I started thinking about you.

I know it sounds like a cliche, but these six years were like a dream. But it wasn't a dream: I didn't imagine them, I lived them and believe me when I say that it's a thousand times better to live your dream than to dream your life! Plus when you dream, you have to wake up sometime. And that's when you realize that your dreams were too enjoyable and that you're back to the realities of everyday life.

Just to say that with your mom, I didn't live six years of lackluster life, but six years of complete felicity.

For our first Christmas, she gave me a mug, and I still use it for my two cups of coffee in the morning. "*Happy to be students*" was what was written on it. That saying corresponded to us well, though we could have said "*Happy to be in love.*" How to describe this love without using commonplace stuff like we always read in novels or see at the movies? Like "*Love Story*?" Did you see it? Our own love story was like a mixture of all of this stuff, but first and foremost, little things, little words we whispered, little things we did, day after day, though sometimes flamboyant ones, as if Jules Verne could have invented them!

We went to the university together, your mom was majoring in French Lit and I was trying my best to graduate as an engineer in microtechnology. She loved words, I loved math. How many times did I say jokingly to her that her French Lit that she saw as "modern" stunk of mothballs and the future of the entire world depended on new technologies and nanotechnologies. When I started talking with these impassioned monologues, she always let me catch my breath, took me by the shoulders, looked me right in the eye and invariably said the same thing.

"Darling, but that's not the future at all! The future is you, me and the kids we'll have together, the future is Love for one another and for those on Earth who don't have enough of it."

I could never trump an answer like that, convinced by her innate goodness. I always let her kiss me and then one thing would lead to another, snuggled in bed.

All these years in college were made of jokes, hugs, just enough studying to graduate… which we both did in the same year.

Then next September, your mom got a job as a French teacher in a middle school in Besancon. And I started doing internships in some big companies based in Switzerland.

The years that followed were each happier than the previous ones. Right up till we decided to start a family. That's when things started to go downhill, as opposed to what you'd be expecting for a project like this.

To make a long story short and perhaps get away from this atmosphere that was weighing both of us down, I said I'd replace one of my colleagues who was sick for a one-week business trip to Milan. It was to negotiate the sale of our newest machines to a whole bunch of industrialists. I was an engineer, replacing a sales guy, so I thought that might help unwind me as I'd have appointment after appointment and all sorts of negotiations which would be tough. The operations manager was aware of this, though he didn't realize he'd be putting salt on my wounds.

"It's not going to be easy Sacha. Those people in Milan, you have to get their checks even if you have to use a pair of *forceps* for the *delivery!*"

Then he tapped me on my shoulder, without noticing my frown that twisted my face with these gynecological terms!

"We're all counting on you!"

When his secretary handed me the plane tickets for Milan, a Friday-to-Friday round trip, I was far from imagining how this would overturn my life... and my family's too, at the same time.

17

Noemie's diary

March, 1987

I FINALLY CALLED DR. *Lepic. When I left her office three months ago, I'd felt so much better. I'd immediately called Sacha and begged him to go on a long vacation, far away, for a month, and without paying any attention to how much this would cost us. After all, and maybe - at least that was what we would be hoping - it would be our last vacation without any children. So might as well take advantage of it before the joy of having kids would change our lives.*

The following Saturday we went to a travel agency and we both fell in love with a tour of the Far West in the States!

A three-week trip winding through the red deserts, flying above the Grand Canyon in a helicopter, wasting a few bucks in the slots in Las Vegas - and to go in whole hog - getting remarried in a fake religious service for twenty dollars, celebrated by a mock priest stuck for the whole day in a hut as small as a toll booth! The opposite of Love: getting married in a drive-in as if you were picking up your order of burgers and fries!

As for accommodations, we had a furnished van: kitchenette, living room, bunks, bathroom, chemical toilet, and a TV antenna.

These three weeks got our minds off our baby-making thoughts, with a total change of scenery. The landscapes, climate, language, nothing brought us mentally back to our existential apprehensions. We made love several times in this little mobile home, naturally, without thinking, attracted to each other only by the purest sensual desires. Pure pleasure, spurred by thoughtless torrid afternoons on vacation.

The last two days though weren't as passionate. We knew our vacation was winding to an end, that we'd quickly have to hop on the plane, land back in France, go home, open the shutters, the gas, do loads and loads of laundry, open our emails, go back to work and our inevitable routines, all our habits, including trying to get pregnant, as ironically I got my period the day the plane landed.

The following weeks weren't much better. Despite frequent intercourse, every two or three days, except for the week that Sacha went to Milan on his trip, nothing happened. That was why I finally decided to pick up my phone and dial Dr. Lepic.

A week later I spread my legs again and slipped my feet into the footrests the peculiar chair that all women fear and all men dream about! The doctor wanted Sacha to be there so we could decide what to do - she had spoken of doing a family history to be exact - so she could decide on what other exams to do later.

So we had to answer loads of questions on our sexual habits, what we ate, any long-term medical treatments, our family's medical history - had anyone had twins, still-borne children, was anyone sterile? - a thorough interrogation, often indiscreet, but something that wasn't actually embarrassing as it was a doctor asking these questions tactfully. Out of the two of us, Sacha was, of course, the one who found it difficult. But it was his first gynecology appointment after all!

After all these questions, she convinced us to undergo further exams to see if one of us, or both of us were suffering from infertility. What an awful word! Not quite as traumatic as "sterility" which seemed more permanent.

And then she continued with a myriad of unnerving medical terms - endoscopy, seminogram, echohysterography, endometriosis - and I'm not even writing the ones I can't pronounce!

"Just routine exams," Dr. Lepic said. "No need to worry about this, just think of them as a checkup! To make sure everything is working... even though Mother Nature is sometimes capricious and wants some couples to take their time."

She filled out several prescriptions.

"Call the gynecology ward in Saint-Jacques Hospital."

Three months before, I had left her office alone, full of hope. This time Sacha and I came out together, but with heavy hearts and knotted stomachs... for the lack of an embryo! One that was full of heartache rather than love.

Chapter 18

Besançon, June, 2015

LEO WAS proud of being the fruit of parents so determined to conceive. Parents forced to take medical tests instead of letting nature take its course. Parents who had to sacrifice an ideal to be forced to undergo dehumanizing machines, reducing a man and a woman whose only hope was to "miraculously" give life to a new human being to two commonplace genitors. Leo suddenly realized that when they both left Dr. Lepic's office, the "miracle of life" no longer existed for them. It would not be a miracle that medicine, despite its power, could ever give them.

Chapter 19

Besançon, May, 1987

NOEMIE WAS in the building's front entrance, leading onto one of the old city's busiest roads. She carefully looked right and left, making sure she didn't see anyone she knew and who could say that she was there. She wasn't far from the school where she worked, students were always walking down this pedestrian road, having a sandwich and listening to music on their Walkmans. Sometimes her colleagues were there too, either window shopping or having lunch out.

She felt guilty, she felt ashamed.

She wasn't sure that she'd made the right decision when she decided to come. She felt bad for having betrayed Sacha, but she couldn't help herself. After all, she also had the right to be selfish, to feel good.

She had finally given in, after much dithering: temptation was too strong, her desire was too powerful. She'd wanted this first appointment, despite the consequences that it could have for their couple.

She didn't know if she'd see him again, if she was strong enough. It was both good and painful. She felt free and guilty at the same time.

Would she be brave enough to tell Sacha about this? Would she be a coward and hide it?

She was weighing the pros and cons of this decision.

Nonetheless, should she never see him again, perhaps it would be better for Sacha if he didn't know?

At the end of the day, it would have been nothing else than a slight mistake, a misdirection, a getaway with no tomorrow.

Her head lowered, she walked down Rue des Granges, examining her options, over and over again, without being able to decide.

Should she give herself a bit more time? The voice of reason.

Then she saw a phone booth at the corner of the road and suddenly wanted to call Aline to ask her. Her best friend would surely be able to give her some good advice. At this time of day she was certainly at home, correcting her papers.

She picked up at the fourth ring.

...

"Aline? It's me, Noe. Am I bothering you?"

...

"That's sweet of you. There's something I wanted to talk to you about."

...

"Yeah, I saw him, and I just got out."

...

"You know, we talked about that. I finally gave in."

...

"I don't know yet. But I must say it did me good."

...

"But here's the problem, I don't know if it's a good idea to see him again. He said it was up to me, that I should decide based on what I want, and also to think about Sacha."

...

"No, I can't tell him. It would be too painful. I'm afraid, you know."

...

"So what would you do? Have you already betrayed Serge?"

...

"Ah, I see... the secret world of women! But if I keep on seeing him, I don't know how I could hide it from Sacha. He'll end up finding out: he knows how to read me, and I don't think I can keep this to myself. Maybe it's better for me to stop while I still have time, before I get hooked on him!"

...

"You know how to talk to me Alinette, thanks. Want to come into town? We could share a cup of hot chocolate?"

...

"Great! You're the best. We can meet at the coffee shop Place de la Revolution. Thanks."

She hung up, dried a little tear in the corner of her eye and went out of the phone booth, feeling a bit less guilty.

20

Noemie's diary

October, 1987

DURING OUR LUNCH BREAK, *I took the car and drove up to the top of Fort de Chadanne, this structure designed by Vauban that overlooks Besancon and gives a great panorama of our city. From up so high you see all four directions without getting tired. You could see all three eras of this Franche-Comté capital: the Citadelle, the Bregille or Griffon Forts, dating back to Vauban; the old city - in the heart of the loop made by the winding and peaceful Doubs River - with its red tiled roofs; and then the soulless buildings, contemporary ones surrounding the old city, spread for over five miles from Chateaufarine up to Chalezeule.*

Anyway, enough of my guided visit! Each time I'm feeling down and it's nice out, I like coming up here in the Fort to look at this urban landscape, observe the branches of the trees waving in the wind or read a few pages of a book to get me thinking of something more positive. And that noon, I had to distance myself from the events so I wouldn't sink into the mental clouding of the past few days.

I was able to relax for a few minutes, empty my head. A few minutes without thinking about those obsessive images haunting me day and night. For a mid-October day, it was really nice: blue sky, warm weather, a slight breeze blowing a few strands of my hair from my bun. Two other people - a couple - must have had the same idea as I did. Everything was there for a few minutes of relaxation before going back to school.

Very quickly though, my demons caught up with me!

It's hard to imagine how the same scene, the same landscapes, the same people or events can be experienced totally differently according to your frame of mind or psychological situation.

I could have noticed beautiful things on this fall day, a couple obviously in love, in this peaceful city, in these historic monuments!

I could have plunged into this novel that I'd been reading for the past couple of days.

Instead of that though, I started to think about time going by, about the seasons. I realized that pregnancy corresponded to three seasons and now it was over a year and a half that we'd been trying to conceive! Two complete cycles of vegetal life had gone by without me being able to feel anything growing inside me!

I was also overlooking the Saint-Jacques Hospital's maternity ward. How many women would be giving birth today beneath my powerless eyes? And how many couples in the population of a hundred and twenty thousand, sleeping under the city's countless roofs, would conceive a child tonight? And how many would accidentally become parents, "victims" of a leaking rubber?

I also felt that this yellow oak leaf that fell from its branch, turning before ending up between the pages of my book, was a bad omen. And if our project were simply a reflection of this dead leaf, one that would always be in the autumn of its life? Or our desire to have a child was fading away also? My stomach was frozen like in winter? When would spring come? And the heat of summer in my intimate organism? And would Dr. Lepic's tests be useful?

Plus I was still up in debate here with my conscience.

I finally decided to see HIM again... and not tell Sacha. He wouldn't understand.

I'm ashamed to admit it, but HE does me good. I have to get away to unwind. Even though, each time I'm with HIM, I cry. But I can see that he's listening, understands me and supports me in his way.

I'm making progress with HIM, but that's what HE'S there for, it was our moral contract as of the very beginning.

We'd decided to see each other again tomorrow at lunch. And I'm actually looking forward to it!

Chapter 21

Besançon, June, 2015

LEO DROPPED his mother's diary as if it had been on fire.

"Jesus!" he exclaimed. "I don't believe it. Have a look at this."

He handed the diary to Chloe.

"Read the last paragraph and tell me what you think." She took a few seconds to read the last lines.

"Do you think she had a lover? I mean like... she was seeing someone?"

"It's something I never could have imagined. You don't have to be a fortune teller to read between the lines: generally speaking when a woman writes HIM in caps in her diary. I can't believe it! A couple who seemed so close, so in love.

I never would have thought my mom could cheat on my dad."

Chloe sat down next to Leo.

"Well, you know, like your dad said when he quoted Sardou: nothing is either all black or white."

"Yeah, now I understand better what he was trying to tell me. Maybe he knew."

"You know, you have to put things back in their context. You've got a couple, seemingly close and in love, but who are going through a long, painful experience, because it's so intimate, it's so important: having a child together. And then months go by, nothing happens, not a glint of hope. So they start doubting, accompanied by bitterness, jealousy and despondency. I think they had two options here: either growing closer because of this failure and getting stronger or their love crumbles away. And then there's an opportunity to get away from it all: an unknown person, someone new, someone surprising, who spices things up. I understand her here."

That however was not what Leo wanted to hear.

"You really think that mom... No."

"It's a human reaction. But look at it this way: at the end of the day, you were born, their couple remained together, in spite of the storms, because it was strong."

"What do you mean? That because of me they stayed together? That if I hadn't been born, they would have split?"

"I don't know, you have to keep on reading, I would imagine that your mom wrote about that too."

Chapter 22

Besançon, June, 2015

THERE WERE videos of planes taking off, one after another, from left to right, right to left, shot from the back or the front, on Leo's PC, while he was looking at his father's tale. The sounds and images made him convinced that these planes were just a symbol of a page that was turning in his father's life.

∽

SACHA'S CD-ROM

FRIDAY, 6:00 a.m. at Orly. I'm just another passenger, a pawn in life's huge chessboard, a spermatozoid lost in a drop of sperm at the bottom of a rubber that's ready to burst! This was about what I thought when I had to go from the check-in counter to the boarding gate, past the duty-free shops.

The night before, when I took the train to Paris, I hugged your mother for a long time. But I also really wanted to get away, escape our preoccupations for a few days, while at the same time wanted to stay with her, not leave her alone brooding over her dark thoughts. We hadn't explicitly mentioned this, because at this time we were not trying just to focus on it, but we both knew that this business trip came at a bad time... right during ovulation.

While we hugged each other at the station, all of this was said in our silences, in the lump in my throat, in your mother's teary eyes.

I stepped into the train, sat down at my reserved seat next to the window and silently said "*I love you*" through the window, words straight from my heart. "*Not as much as I do*," I lipread from her adorable lips.

Then the train started up... and I was soon in the Alitalia plane taking off!

Just an hour and a half trip from Paris to Milan. Not long, but enough to overturn an existence, enough to shatter your convictions and to begin an unexpected human adventure... I had time to experience all of that while I was flying over the Alps at 30,000 feet. And this, my dear son, this key moment of my life, I owe it to you to describe it as well as I can.

Everything was the result of a commonplace incident. The plane had just reached its cruise altitude and the flight attendants had started serving breakfast: the traditional little plastic tray with a roll, a carton of milk and a mini package of cereals, without forgetting to ask us this inevitable question: *"What would you like? Tea or coffee?"* I asked for a cup of coffee that the attendant, dressed in a suit with Italy's national colors on it, served in a white plastic cup. After that, I often thought about this very second offering us a malicious fate. Had the plane not experienced turbulence at that very same second, I never would have even glanced at this lady while taking my hot cup of coffee from her. But the plane suddenly dropped, the flight attendant lost her balance for a second, the cup flying out of her hands and landing on my white shirt!

She told me how very sorry she was with that cute Transalpine accent.

"I'm so sorry, *signor*, please follow me and we'll get that washed up."

I looked up from my "coffee-white" shirt, began to complain, but then I saw her for the first time.

A slight digression here!

Remember when I told you that it was love at first sight when I met your beautiful mom and I told you that it was something you only experienced once in a lifetime? Well, I still think so! Of course, that's something that only happens once! But here I'm telling you this, that day in the plane, when my eyes met those of the Italian flight attendant, I swear to God it was like "lightning struck!"

Lightning, it's so bright, it lights up your life. Thunder... it deafens you, it makes you blind to reason, it fills your ears and brain with a sound you can't get rid of.

At the movies or in books, they try to make us believe we can be lost in someone's eyes. But on the contrary, I thought I was found!

"Don't worry, it's not a big deal," I finally answered, putting an end to this silence while we stared into each other's eyes.

She invited me to follow her to the back of the plane to "fix it."

"My *nonna*, I mean my grandma, always said that for a coffee stain, you had to use vinegar water or warm water with an egg yolk."

I had already quit listening to her though.

I was drinking her in, better than the coffee I didn't have!

She was dabbing the stain with paper towels. But all I could see was her curly hair pulled back in a bun (hygiene I guess)!

"I do apologize," she kept on saying, while trying to get the stain out.

"It's not a problem. Just tell me your name."

"Maeva."

"I love it!"

We stood very close to one another in this tiny space between the refrigerators, heat blocs and chemical toilets, pushed towards each other by the plane's continued turbulence. We were alone, the remainder of the personnel were still serving breakfast.

"I'm Sacha," I continued. "I'll be in Milan for a week on business. Would you accept an invitation to have a drink one of these days if you're in Milan? So I can forgive you!"

"I don't know, I..."

I didn't let her finish. I just gave her my business card after I'd written down the address of the hotel I'd be staying in.

"Give me a call."

And then I went back to my seat, leaving her alone with my audacious invitation.

When the plane stopped at its gangway, all the passengers, whether they were looking forward to their business appointments or seeing their loved ones again, swarmed up to the front to rush out. I deliberately took my good old-fashioned time to put my jacket back on and put my book away before opening the overhead to get my carry-on. I was thus the last one out and while leaving the plane, I looked deep in Maeva's eyes once again, thinking of the turbulence that was at the origin of our meeting just a few minutes ago and who I already couldn't stop thinking of.

"Have a nice stay in Milan," she politely and conventionally said.

"I'm sure it will be enchanting," I mysteriously answered, without looking away from her.

Then I disappeared in the intestines of the gangway without turning around, to be sure I wouldn't be able to see if she was still looking at me.

WHEN I GOT to my nice little room in the Starhôtels Rosa, a sophisticated venue located right in the middle of the city near the famous Duomo, I unpacked, got undressed and took a long hot shower to clear my mind.

And while the water was streaming down over my closed eyes, my mind didn't clear at all. Quite the contrary. What the hell had I been thinking of when I flirted with that flight attendant I hadn't even known existed two hours before? Why had I felt that "thunderclap" when looking at her? How can a man who is so in love with his wife and who's only wish is to have a child with her be attracted like this to someone totally unknown? Those were some of the thousands of questions running through my head.

I tried to coldly analyze this event in this hot shower, thinking of the last few months.

First of all it was categorically impossible to

believe that I could have been attracted ferociously by this woman because I was no longer attracted to my wife! My wife - your mother, son - has always attracted me, and at that time, not less than when I first met her.

So, what? Why had I felt this instinctive need of someone exotic? Was it a mere game? What was I really expecting here? Was I hoping to find a new love, stronger than my old one, or just a one-night stand, far from my daily life, or even just a good time having a glass of something in a bar in Milan, in good company, without any hidden agendas other than being nice?

Or maybe all of it at the same time?

Whatever the reason, I was no longer pulling the strings. Maeva was the one who would decide whether or not to come. I'd handed her a business card, it was up to her whether to give me a call or throw the card away, forget this unknown person who must not have been the first one to try to get to know her better and just continue on with her life as if nothing had happened in the plane, as if our eyes had never sparkled with that troubling glint when we first looked at each other.

All I knew was her first name and the persistent image on my retina.

I was suddenly dizzy. Was it this situation or was the water too hot?

Would she even call?

I was starting to have my doubts. Had she

thought I was a fruitcake or a mid-life crisis serial flirt who couldn't help himself each time he saw a beautiful prey? I realized that in her line of work, she must meet at least one per flight, these guys with a gift of gab who try to hook up far from their little lady's back at home.

Yes, Maeva must have had her fill of guys like me! Until she was sick and tired of it, though she would continue to smile with her white teeth while pouring you a glass of wine, wishing you a good stay when you were leaving the plane, as she must have been taught to do, always so professionally.

While I was drying off, I had reached the conclusion that she'd never call me and that was probably a good thing...

... until the phone rang.

I picked up, a bit nervous, and the hotel clerk told me I had a message at the front desk. I quickly got dressed and rushed down.

"How about a drink tonight at Giancarlo's?" was what was written.

"I'd like to answer please."

He handed me a form to fill in.

"Va bene!" I wrote, exhausting my few words of Italian.

That whole day, between two appointments with automobile outsourcers, all I could think of were two faces: your mom's and hers. I saw them like in cartoons when someone is hesitating between two alternatives: a little angel on one side telling you to do the right thing and a little devil on the other, spurring you to do the opposite.

I felt like I was on top of a gigantic slide, ready to let go and slide down the slope that would lead me to a huge mistake!

Chapter 23

Besançon, June, 2015

LEO AND CHLOE were sitting on a bench in Micaud Park, holding hands, peacefully watching the river that found its source in the Haut-Doubs plateau and wound itself around the base of the Citadelle.

They'd decided to take a break after having watched this part of Sacha's surprising CD-ROM. They couldn't get it out of their minds.

"This has gone from bad to worse," said Leo. "What else will they be telling me? I don't know if I want to find out more. I'm afraid to read or hear things that are really none of my business."

"Well, you can stop now, you know. No one will criticize you if you don't want to learn anymore."

"Sure! But it is pretty tempting, I must admit.

Even if I'm going to find out that they cheated on each other: first my mom, then my dad."

"You're getting ahead of yourself here. How do you know that your dad and that Italian actually did it? We have no idea at this point."

And it was true that a few moments ago, Leo had slammed his finger on the pause button so he wouldn't hear anymore. Then he'd ejected the CD-ROM, ready to toss it in the bin under his desk. Chloe had stopped him, gently putting her hand on his.

"Don't do that, it's something they left you. You can ignore it, but not destroy it. Who knows? Maybe, one day you'll come back to it."

"I really like this park," Leo said, quickly changing the subject. "We often came here when I was little. I went to Helvetie School, right next to it. My dad always took me on the merry-go-round, right next to it. They updated it, but it's still in the same place. Plus I liked running after the ducks on the riverbanks. Sometimes we played soccer too. And on Sundays sometimes, the three of us had picnics here: we'd put our stuff down on a red and white checkered tablecloth on the lawn overlooking the river."

A bittersweet tear welled up in Leo's already red eye. The young man's face was tired, marked by insomnia in the past few nights, grieving during the days, memories of the past and the *post-mortem* revelations of his parents.

"Enough with all this," Chloe said. "Let's go eat in a nice little restaurant in town. Which one do you want to go to?"

"I don't know, something simple. How about the Brasserie du Commerce?"

"Fine with me! It's a real cute one." Turning talk into action, they left the park, their arms around one another. They crossed the Doubs, took the Republique Bridge to Revolution Square, where a few decades ago, Grigor Kapinsky, Leo's maternal grandfather, used to teach at the Conservatory of Music.

Chapter 24

Besançon, April 11, 1987

THEY WALKED out of Camponovo Bookshop, on Grande Rue, each one holding a new novel. They both needed to intellectually escape for a couple of hours. Sacha had purchased *It* by Stephen King: he liked this author who knew how to draw on everyone's primeval fears, those when you were little. Noemie liked true stories much better, and had been attracted by Dominique Lapierre's book, *The City of Joy*, hoping to be consoled by the story: all her little problems were nothing at all compared to Calcutta's huge shantytowns.

Noemie took Sacha's hand while they were aimlessly walking down the pedestrian street that afternoon. Then she stopped.

"Did you like Milan? Did you have time to tour the city a little?"

Sacha was a bit taken aback by her sudden question.

"Yeah, a little. But you know I spent most of my time with customers. It was a huge contract. There were lots of machines to calibrate, lots of Italian engineers to train, projects to be finalized. All that stuff, you know!"

"Well, to be honest, I actually don't. I'm sure your job must be really interesting, I'm not saying it's not and I can see you really like it, but it's not my thing. I can't imagine it, it seems too complex to me. My job is easier to describe, isn't it?"

"Sure, everyone had teachers in their life! But not sales engineers in micro-technologies."

"You must be tired then. Did you have time to go out?" she continued.

"I had to!" Sacha replied nervously. "I had to take my customers out. Really boring: expensive restaurants, everyone wearing a suit and tie, drinking wine. In theory, really nice, but in reality, really tiring and difficult."

"Oh! Sweetie! You did come home really tired. Those Italians wore you out. Did you go to a nightclub?"

"Why are you asking me that?" Sacha said nervously, feeling more and more uncomfortable.

"Why all these questions?" he thought. *And how come she's suddenly so interested in my job? Does she suspect some-*

thing? Plus the night club question. Did she find something in one of my pockets? Or smell something? That must be it, women know how to smell other women. Or maybe a strand of Maeva's hair on one of my jackets?"

"Hello, this is Earth calling," said Noemie, cutting off his line of thought.

"Ah! Excuse me, um no, we didn't go to any night clubs. But Italians live at night and the restaurants are all open really late."

"And is it a nice city? It makes me think of something all grey and industrial, full of pollution."

"Actually that's what I thought too. But the city center is old and charming. Not as beautiful as Florence or Rome, but it does look like a nice place to live."

"And you have to go back?"

Mental images of seeing Milan... and Maeva once again were invading Sacha's brain. He was wondering if she could see it in his eyes as they must have been twinkling.

"Probably once a month or every two months, at least at first."

Noemie was immediately interested by this response.

"Hey, if it's during school vacation, maybe I could come with you? Would that be possible? That would be awesome, for the seventh anniversary of when we first met."

"Is she doing it on purpose? Trying to test me? See how I react? Trick me?"

"Sure, I think it would be possible. There's no reason why my employer would forbid me from doing what I want during my free time. Like I don't work 24/7 for him! Plus there's a double bed in the hotel!"

She rested her head on Sacha's shoulder, dreaming.

"Italy. I've never been there but everyone loves it. What about the Italian women - are they as beautiful as they say too? Sophia Loren, Ornella Muti, Gina Lollobrigida…"

Sacha burst out laughing.

"Haha! They're movie stars. I can reassure you that I saw more Mammas wearing aprons, smoking cigarettes and carrying a rolling pin with them than divas!"

"Yeah sure, good try mister!" All the color left Sacha's face.

"What do you think I'm hiding?"

"I don't know. Like a good-looking guy like you, on a business trip abroad, far from his wife..."

"Stop it now, you're imagining things. You know I love you honey."

"Really? "No, I didn't," she said, making fun of him. "Repeat it once."

"I love you."

Noemie stood up on her tiptoes and kissed him.

"I love you too."

And they continued their walk, hand-in-hand,

stopping to window shop, sometimes going in, buying little trinkets.

Sacha suddenly realized what time it was.

"Shoot, I almost forgot I had squash at five with Loic. I'm going to have to be going. What are you going to do?"

THIS TIME NOEMIE didn't know what to say to Sacha. She did know however what she'd planned to do! She just hadn't thought that she'd have to tell him what she'd be doing from five to seven. Meaning she didn't have an alibi at the tip of her tongue. She tried to wiggle out of the question.

"I don't know yet. How long are you going to play?" Noemie knew quite well what she was going to do. She was just trying to gain some time.

"About an hour. After that, a good hot shower with Lolo, and how about we meet here again in two hours? That okay for you?"

Noemie quickly did her math: generally speaking when she saw HIM, they would spend an hour together, an intense one. After that she'd rush back home, put on new makeup and erase all traces of the emotional havoc wreaked by this stolen hour, this secret hour, with this mysterious man she was afraid to tell Sacha about.

She still felt guilty about betraying Sacha like that. Yet she loved him. That's why she didn't want to risk hurting him by telling him about this.

Perhaps, later on, she wouldn't need to see HIM again. Perhaps she'd forget all of that and it would just be a short story to bury in her secret world. He'd never know and that would be a good thing!"

"Sure," she said, coming out of her thoughts. "Seven o'clock here."

"Fine. You going back home?" Sacha asked again.

"Um no. I think I'll hang around in town some more. Or maybe go see Aline. Serge works in the garage on Saturdays, so maybe I'll stop by for a cup of tea."

They then each went their own way, both interiorizing their own lies, what was unsaid and their subconscious suspicions.

Two hours later, they met at the Brasserie du Commerce to enjoy a meal in the well-conserved 19th century building with its high ceilings.

Chapter 25

Besançon, June, 2015

WHEN LEO and Chloe left the Brasserie du Commerce, night had already fallen, just like the scruples of the young man to continue looking at the CD-ROM his father had left him.

That was all they had talked about while eating and Chloe had convinced him that he had to pay tribute to his father's memory by listening to all of his confessions. Even if that would mean hearing difficult things. As soon as they got back to their apartment, Leo immediately put the CD back into his laptop.

∾

SACHA'S CD-ROM

Milan, April 3, 1987

SO WHY AM I telling you all this? You must be wondering why I want you to know the sordid details of this extra-marital affair. But please, and here I'm begging you, don't judge me before you know the end of this story. Everything that you're hearing and seeing now has always remained hidden deep down inside, amongst all the other unholy things that make up the lives of human beings. I have to get it out and you're the only one who can receive this confession!

That night we met in a trendy bar, the *TriBeCa Lounge*, near the banks of the *Niviglo Pavese*, this canal linking Milan to Pavie, that goes through the city and gives both its inhabitants and tourists the opportunity of enjoying a cocktail or coffee while dipping their toes into the water. Like you'd see on a postcard.

"I wasn't expecting such a nice city," I began, so I wouldn't give her the impression of someone as silent as the grave, while being totally in awe of Maeva's beauty and charisma.

"That's exactly what most tourists say when they first come here," she answered, in her beautiful voice, half sophisticated and half throaty, a crackly voice we imagine all Italians have.

See Leo, I was completely spellbound by her Transalpine beauty. I continued.

"I'd thought of Milan as being a dark and smokey industrial city. And I naively had imagined rows and rows of houses for those working for Fiat! Like Italian miners!

"You must have read Germinal too much! *Bene*, but that's what most people think. If you want, I can show you around the romantic part of Milan."

"Well, with a guide like you, how could I refuse!"

"Flattery will get you nowhere, Sacha."

She looked me straight in the eyes. It was unsettling. I had no answer to that and she continued.

"Do you like to have a good time, dance, drink, or sing?"

"Don't forget I'm here for business!"

"Well. It's up to you! I've got a tour that you'll love. Ever heard of *La Dolce Vita*?

"Ah! Mastroianni..."

"No, no, I'm not talking about Fellini's movie here, I'm talking about the true *Dolce Vita*, the *Navigli*, *Sempione* Park, the *Piazza Mercanti*, the *Pinacotheque*, happy hours in the bars, enjoying steaming *latte machhiato* on Sunday afternoons! All these little things that make Milan a mixture of Renaissance and modernity."

"You're talking about Sunday, does that mean that your program also includes Saturday night?

"You're perceptive, Sherlock Sacha!" (And always with this captivating look and enchanting smile at the end of each of her sentences.) "But don't forget that tonight it's Friday and they also serve brunch on Saturday."

"If I understand you correctly, I'm your hostage as of tonight? The party is going to start now?"

"It's already started," she added with a smile and dipped her pulpy lips into her glass of *Martini Rosso*.

I didn't believe it! Such self-assurance! She was showing me who the boss really was, with finesse, but directly. After all, I was the one who kicked this off in the plane, and I couldn't complain here about being shaken up by her.

We had another round of drinks and kept on talking. Now Maeva was having a *Martini Bianco*.

"First a *Rosso*, then a *Bianco*. It's a tradition in our family.

I was having another *Negroni*, a common cocktail made from *Martini Rosso*, *Bitter Campari*, gin and served on the rocks. A tad aggressive, but it hit the spot.

As the cocktails and appetizers whet another appetite than carnal, we decided to walk along the banks after happy hour, changing venues.

It was still nice out at that time on the bank of the *Naviglo Pavese* that we took to walk to Magenta, one of Milan's most popular restaurants. I think Maeva must have been trying to impress me by choosing the most trendy and romantic places in Milan.

And she did!

She must have been a regular here. I could tell that she knew the waiter who seated us.

"There is always a table for *una bella ragazza* like you *Signorina*," he said, showing us to a table in an isolated corner of the restaurant.

"Let me order for you," my delicious flight attendant suggested. "I'll guide your taste buds towards culinary pleasures that you've never even imagined."

"Just culinary pleasures?" I asked.

"We'll start with culinary ones, *Signor* Sacha."

So she ordered typical Milan dishes for us. And all I had imagined were Milan-style veal scallops! Instead of that, I discovered *risotto a la milanese* prepared with bouillon and beef marrow for our antipasti, then we had *vitello tonnait*, a delicious slice of veal in sauce made from tuna, mayonnaise, anchovies and capers. And to wash it all down, a bottle of *Barbera dell'Oltrepo Pavese*.

Such a surprising city. Discoveries leading to astonishment, following my Italian flight attendant's judicious suggestions, as even on the ground, she remained welcoming, smiling and so very seductive!

Our meal was succulent, our conversation delicious.

We started out with pleasant small talk. Both of us seemed to feel that this evening could only be a magical interlude for us, so we didn't talk about our lives, our past, all the things that could destroy this atmosphere in the snap of two fingers!

Some incorrigible flirts swear by the "pity me" technique. That's when they talk about their aches and pains and mistakes they made in the past to give them the key to the prey of the moment's heart and bed.

With Maeva we unconsciously preferred to laugh, talk joyfully, take advantage of that moment, enjoy the nice music being played in the *trattoria*, as well as the flavors and various odors of our meals.

I could feel that she was an Epicurean in her life, I shared that point of view. I was fulfilled by her beauty, my other senses by this charming little restaurant. All that was missing was the sense of touch! But I was expecting that it would soon follow...

～

NOW THAT I'M telling you this, I feel ashamed. I remember that during this entire evening, at no moment whatsoever did I think about your mother. I was so subjugated by this Italian that I forgot everything else: my business trip, my own wife, our omnipresent difficulties we were having to conceive. For one evening, all that became something like a watermarked image, an unconscious souvenir way in the background of the present moment. Yet I would have had a thousand reasons to worry about your mother, alone at home. Alone with her apprehension that she'd never be a mother, alone with the months we spent not being able to give life.

Instead of that, I selfishly enjoyed these exotic pleasures given to me, and did this the very first time that I'd been alone for a couple of days and nights, away from home.

You could say that this business trip had turned into an outlet for all the stress I'd accumulated the past few months. I ran without looking towards a one-night-stand, a sensual escape that I was already thinking of as a homeopathic remedy.

Remedy or hospice care?

Would this adventure cure me of my apprehension or just push it back?

When I'd get back from Milan, would I be cured of my negative mood, or would I sink even deeper into this ocean of pessimism? Whatever, those were not questions I was asking myself that evening, I was living in the moment!

Maeva had called a cab for us.

"Buona sera, signor. Al Hollywood per favore."

"What, from Milan to Hollywood in a cab? That's going to cost a bundle."

"You didn't review your Milan classics before disembarking, *caro Sacha*! Hollywood is Milan's and even Lombardy's most famous nightclub! Maybe even Italy's most famous one!"

"Must be hard to get in then."

"Perhaps you've noticed that I get in wherever I

want. I know a lot of people. Traveling first class, that helps."

"Including bouncers?"

"Especially them."

"*Allons danser alors*," I whispered to her, taking her hand on the back seat of the cab.

Indeed, getting in was a piece of cake for us. They showed us to an alcove, a bit away from the dance floor, where a few other people were already seated. Two men and two women. One of them jumped up from the couch as soon as he saw Maeva and began speaking Italian style with his hands.

"*Ma que bella Maeva!*"

He air-kissed her on both cheeks while running his fingers through her hair. She looked back at me.

"This is Luca Giordano, one of Milan's leading fashion designers. Luca, this is Sacha, someone I was lucky to have met on the plane."

We had to speak loudly to be heard above the loud metallic music. We ordered a bottle of whisky and Coke, like everyone else in night clubs everywhere.

I met the others. There was Giustina, a mannequin at Elite who followed Luca everywhere. The other couple was Virginia, an actress in series B movies in Hollywood (the real one this time!) and Franco M., a well-known politician. This apparently was the place to be for anyone who was anything in Milan or in Italy for that matter, the place where you had to be seen. Maeva, a mere Alitalia flight attendant, must have been the most ordinary person in this nocturnal fauna. Yet she seemed so at ease and seemed to know most of the people there. How well did she know them? Just people she'd met while she was out? Or did she have more intimate links with these politicians, artists, or businessmen? Whatever, most of the people we saw seemed to be happy to see her. I was starting to get a bit jealous though I'd only known her for a few hours! How should I interpret this feeling? Was I falling in love or just suffering from the vaguely animal like reflex of a tiger in its cage with other felines trying to seduce the most beautiful female tiger in the group? Who'd win? How to make the female notice you? How to be the leader of the pack?

Luca brought me back from this daydreaming.

"Have you known Maeva long?"

"Just a few hours."

"Well, you sure made an impression on her! I know her well and I saw it right away!"

He spoke like stylists all over the world do, with a high voice, unexpected intonations, and exaggerated gestures. Like a mixture of Karl Lagerfeld, Jean-Paul Gaultier and Giorgio Armani - for his Transalpine accent - when he made the effort to speak French to me.

"Can I give you some advice as a friend, Sacha?"

"I'm listening."

"Don't get too close to this *ragazza*. She'll make

you suffer horribly. Take it from someone who's been there! Maeva eats men alive! If she takes one little nibble, you'll be lost forever."

"*Mamma mia!*"

Raising his glass of whisky-Coke, he laughed out loud and held out his glass to me.

"Here's to you, Sacha!"

No need to add anything else, I got it.

We both looked over to the dance floor where Maeva stood out in a group mainly composed of males in heat. Her splendid body was writhing from right to left, from top to bottom with the music. Her center of gravity must have been located in the hollow of her back which was rocking in a totally hypnotic spiral while her slim fingers were running through her long wavy hair. Like the whole evening was concentrated around her buttocks that seemed to be calling out to me! In the past few hours, I felt as if I had been sucked into a cyclone, or the little whirlwind that you see when you empty out the tub: concentric circles that lure you into the eye of the cyclone and there's nothing at all you can do about it. That's how, without even noticing it (perhaps inebriated by the noise and alcohol), I found myself on the dance floor too, rubbing up against Maeva's back, swaying in the same rhythm as she was, my hands on her thighs, lifting her skirt, my sex hard against her rear...

Like I was a part of her, like nothing else existed around us. I sought out her nape hidden by her hair to kiss it, to drink in her perfume and the sugary taste of her hot skin.

A few seconds later (or maybe a few hours, I had no idea), my body dominated hers on a comfy couch. My hands ran against her curves looking for happiness, my tongue went deep into her mouth in the hopes of finding a drop of her precious nectar.

I was in the eye of the cyclone. The tipping point. This time, nothing around us existed anymore: neither the nightclub, nor our desire to have children, nor Noemie (that's awful!), nor Maeva herself, nor me...

Chapter 26

Saint-Gothard Tunnel, February, 2015

IT TOOK Pippo about four hours to reach the Saint-Gothard Tunnel, with the steep slopes in the highways in the Alps and Swiss customs to go through.

But he was far from having finished. Now his truck was in line behind loads of others, waiting to enter the seventeen kilometers of the tunnel going through the mountain.

In 2001, a Belgian truck had run head-on into an Italian truck coming from the opposite direction, setting off a fire where eleven people perished. The driver, a Turk, had had too much to drink and had fallen asleep behind the wheel, and to top it all off, he was working illegally. As he also lost his life, he didn't shed any tears for the ten other innocent victims.

As a consequence of this accident though, rules became much stricter. Now trucks were only allowed to circulate in one direction at a time, leading to interminable lines at the entrance. The price to be paid to avoid new tragedies.

Pippo decided to relax a little, stretch, have a cup of coffee from his thermos, check his emails and messages on his phone, as once in the tunnel, he wouldn't be able to.

Night was beginning to fall. It was after five. Pippo liked to drive at night, if possible, on major highways where there weren't too many vehicles, feeling like a solitary wolf at home in its snow-filled steppes. That's why he liked to deliver goods in the Baltic countries, or in Poland or Ukraine.

He was no longer afraid of the night and its solitude. Not after those ten long years.

He'd been a night owl before that. But always in a good crowd. Surrounded by his friends, by easy women, spotlights and disco balls, inhaling vapors of alcohol and illegal smoke. Lots of money, lots of alcohol, lots of girls. Maybe too many?

Too suddenly, too quickly. All of this had gone to his head, burned his neurons... and his wings.

The Swiss radio blared out in French, German, and Italian, changing his line of thought.

« *The Saint-Gothard Tunnel is still very busy. We'd like to remind our truck-driving friends that they must comply with road space rationing, and we thank them for their patience and their professional conduct. The weather is stationary: a few light snowstorms, but the snow plows are in place to clear the highway. We would like to remind you that you cannot pass trucks while they are spreading salt. And finally, of course Saint-Gothard Peak is closed. Drive safely and be careful. And to accompany you, here's Adèle's latest single, 'Hello.'"*

Pippo loved that song. He turned it up, though it didn't stop him from thinking.

It was true that he had had everything much too quickly. He'd had no idea what to do with all that and lost it all. Because of a woman.

Who he'd been unable to keep, unable to love.

It had been his own fault here, as he'd been too selfish, too focused on himself only, on his ambitions, on his future.

At this time he already had long hair, though he didn't have to attach it into a ponytail, as he'd had nice, curly hair, like most Italians. At that time his knee didn't ache like it did nowadays, especially when it was cold or damp and he had to turn the heat on high in his cab to ease the pain.

That damn knee that reminded him of that bitch. He'd lost both at the same time: the woman and his knee. And that wasn't all.

But now was maybe time for revenge.

But was revenge really what he was dreaming of? Or just revenge on his life?

When he was finally allowed to go into the

tunnel, he thought maliciously that this trip would be the one leading him to his long-awaited revenge.

The truck entered the highway's entrails and disappeared in the mountain.

27

Noemie's diary

January, 1988

BOTH SACHA *and I began our tests. For him, it was much easier. Some bloodwork and a seminogram! That means a sample of the sperm liquid. And I have to admit here that we both cracked up doing it, a comical interlude in the middle of this psychological drama. To make this test less "traumatic," as the secretary in the gynecology ward said with a chuckle, we could do it at home.*

But how?

Did Sacha have to fill up his test tube alone? A solitary and manual job? Did he have to be alone, concentrating on what he was doing, in the bathroom? And to get in the mood, would he have the right to leaf through men's magazines or rent a video by Marc Dorcel that he'd look at in the living room? Or perhaps just think of the lascivious body of his dear wife? We thought about all these possibilities but finally decided to make it a duo. I'd have to help him get in the mood, help that precious sap to be analyzed spring forth...

So that's how we did it!

But then afterwards I thought that perhaps saliva would be detectable in a test tube!

Anyway, it was funny, up until we got the results.

Nothing to report on Sacha's sperm.

So the problem didn't stem from that side, nor in his bloodwork that just said that he'd have to pay attention to his glycemia rates. That should have been reassuring, but it also meant that I was the one who had a problem here. Unless it was an incompatibility between the two of us.

Things were starting to get complicated. Without mentioning ethics, legal matters or psychological impacts, it's easy to understand that if the guy is the one with a problem, the solutions and consequences of artificial insemination aren't as important. Sperm only plays its role for a few minutes or hours. So it's like a medical piece of cake to inseminate sperm from the father or from an anonymous donor. But the chance of success drops when it's the woman who's infertile, as an embryo has to be implanted or oocytes have to be donated. Success falls from seventy-five percent for a man to less than twenty for a woman.

Now that it's time for me to put my positive attitude on, I'm starting to get scared. If I want to improve my chances, Dr. Lepic insists that I have to have a positive mindset.

But I'm getting ahead of myself here.

Let's get all the tests done and get their results first.

MARCH, **1988**

A FEW DAYS of apprehension while waiting for the results.

I can't eat, I can't sleep. I know I'm bitchy with my poor Sacha, something he sure doesn't deserve! I'm the one with the problem and he's the one I'm taking it out on!

I love you Sacha. If you ever read this, I want you to know how sorry I am. But you have to understand, it's my integrity as a woman, a mother, someone who gives life, that's at stake here and I'm completely overwhelmed.

Yet I know that you understand me and for that, once again, I love you.

28

Sacha's CD-ROM

Milan, April 3, 1987

THAT NIGHT, I don't know how, but we ended up in my hotel room. I can't tell you any details, but I can describe what went on in three words: passion, wild, timeless...

Later that morning we called for room-service. Delicious *panettone*.

"Will we be seeing each other again?" I asked, between two bites.

She just sighed.

"Sacha, I loved last night, I loved what we did together, but I'm not capable of building any relationships."

"Of course. I was just wondering."

"You're married though, right?"

How did she know? I'd carefully taken my

wedding ring off, slipping it into my wallet before we'd arrived at the restaurant.

"Wedding rings leave prints on your finger," she continued, as if she could read my mind. "I think it would be better just to leave things as they are. It was fantastic, something I'll never forget, and I don't regret a thing I did or said last night, *caro* Sacha."

"Me neither, I'd do it again... But I love my wife, I can't imagine my life without her."

"Tell me about her."

"You sure?"

"Why do you love her?"

"Vast question there. Who knows why you love one person rather than another? Who can say that they'll only fall in love once? And can you love several women at the same time? And how can you believe that the love of your life is someone you haven't even met? But can you spend your life looking for 'your better half,' as Plato would say? You know that myth?"

"Tell me, I've always loved stories."

"So Plato thought that at the beginning of time, the Creator, furious at men, had literally cut them all in half (at that time men were half men and half women), and that he then spread them all around the Earth. So during their whole lives, each of the parts (male and female) would never stop looking for their 'true carnal half.' Sometimes they found each other and made a perfect whole. But more often than not, they looked but never met, and just created imperfect couples."

"What an incredible theory! That would explain why so many people are frustrated and pathological cheaters! You think your wife is your other half?"

"I don't know. All I know is that she makes me very happy and I don't feel like I'm frustrated living with her. What about you, still looking for your other half?"

"Me?" she said, laughing. "I prefer a thousand times being alone rather than being with the wrong person. I'm as free as a bird, my spirit and body don't have any constraints. I think I'm closer to Epicure than Plato."

"Have you ever been married?"

"Never! Men are a hobby for me. I suffered from their selfishness and brutality. But that's another story…"

She had goosebumps and was frowning unconsciously. I would have liked to know why she was so virulent about marriage, but I was afraid to ask. I didn't want to spark memories that would have spoiled this beautiful sun-filled morning.

She changed subjects.

"Do you have any kids?"

Now it was my turn! Like someone had slugged me in the face. She'd found my skeleton in the closet. But it was like an opportunity for me. I felt that I had to free myself from this heavy weight on my heart and I was thus nearly relieved to be able to talk about this with someone who was not involved and who would lend an attentive ear.

"Not yet, and that's the problem. We've been trying for months now. That's all we think about the whole day and the whole night too. It's like torture for us to want this so badly and not to be able to do anything about it! We've lost taste for everything else; we're obsessed, we even have the impression that we're killing our life as a couple."

"So that's why you escaped into my arms then?"

"Maybe. Just for one night, it was like I was a man again, and not a 'future father.' Just for that I want to thank you."

"My pleasure!"

And she kissed me to punctuate her sentence. She tasted like blueberry jam. I wanted her again. I pushed the breakfast tray away with one hand while caressing her proud and tiny breasts with the other. Then my hand disappeared under the sheets and we made love once again.

꙳

"I'M GOING BACK to Paris tomorrow," she said when leaving. "You've got my number. Call me if you need me. I'll be there."

꙳

SO THAT MY SON, is how I met the second woman in my life. Your mother never knew a thing about her, she was like a flash of lightning in my life. A flash of lighting that struck me and burned me. Now I'll tell you why.

Noemie's diary

April, 1988

RESULTS ARE COMING *in and they seem to be encouraging: my tubes aren't blocked, my ovaries are doing their job, so is my uterus, and I'm not having premature menopause.*

Okay. Great. So what else is new?

If everything's working, what's the problem Doc? Now each time I get some good news it's like it's bad news as nothing seems to be coming of it.

If my tubes had been blocked, at least we could understand!

But they're not! Everything's fine!

Now even the doctors are having doubts, and we're getting desperate!

JULY 15, **1988**

DR. *Lepic is pulling her hair out.*

Weeks are going by, we're undergoing tests, and still nothing. We're an "interesting" case and she's personally going to follow us. We are said to be amongst the six percent of couples who are infertile for an unknown reason.

In accordance with our doctors, we've decided to consult some bigwig in fecundation. Sometimes, the cause can be due to a genetic malformation in the mother or father.

Dr. Lepic gave us a list of specialists in Paris who would be interested in our rare condition.

So now Sacha and I have to make a choice: do we still want to conceive a child? If so, are we ready to undergo, once again, all those many heavy tests?

For the moment, we've decided to think about it before asking for an appointment in Paris.

30

Sacha's CD-ROM

I left Milan three days later and quickly segued back into my daily life. My professional briefcase was full of juicy contracts while my sentimental baggage was both tortured and appeased.

For those three entire days and up till I got back, that was all I could think about. What had I done? What had that one-night-stand brought me? What would I lose? Should I tell Noemie about what I did and if so, would she understand? Or should I put it away in my closet of unholy secrets and make sure she never knew? What would hurt her the most: knowing that I'd cheated on her or my guilty silence, with the possibility that one day she might find out?

Dozens of questions and scenarios were flying around in my head, and I had no idea what to do. At the last minute though, I decided to tell her everything. I was sure she'd forgive me if I confessed. I believed this until I saw her, tears in her eyes, on our front porch.

"I missed you so much my Love."

"Me too, Darling."

"Let's go make a baby!"

I just had the time to put my suitcase down before she pulled me towards her and into the bedroom where she'd lit candles for a romantic atmosphere.

We made love with tears in our eyes. We made love warmly. They were tears of hope.

A pleasure of despair.

When our bodies pulled away, I knew it was too late to say anything. I no longer had enough strength. Only one thing I could think of: loving Noemie and making her the mother of our children. My whole life would be devoted to this goal, and this one only. Everything else was secondary compared to this primordial objective.

In the days after I got back from Italy, I realized something that should have been evident: I was in love with my wife! I mean that I loved her even more than before I'd left for Milan. Or maybe I didn't realize before Milan how much I did love her. Just because I'd left for a few days, I'd made love briefly with someone I'd never met before and my eyes were opened to this reality: maybe my wife wasn't my 'Platonian half' but she was my purpose in life and I had the duty to make her happy. I had had to step back, try something new, to be aware of how happy I really was.

Never forget my dear son: happiness is often just around the corner and you sometimes have to step back to notice it.

I was thus able to unconsciously overlook everything and throw my body and soul into this project that would make us the happiest people in the world in the future: having a baby.

We tried each and every method, we calculated everything imaginable, but without any results. Several months went by, almost a year I think, and during this time we deliberately paused our "make a baby" project so we could clear our minds and not sink into a depression and defeatism that could have destroyed both of us.

I had several business trips to Milan and sometimes met with Maeva. Though I felt guilty each time, I also curiously felt that this woman was going to bring me something, that I'd met her for a reason, as if fate had put her on my road, like a guardian angel for our couple. I know, it's a paradox, but that's what I felt.

Then one day, your mom and I decided to try one more time: I had the contact details of a Parisian specialist who…

THE SCREEN WAS FROZEN on Sacha's face, and he hadn't finished his sentence.

Chapter 31

Saint-Jean-de-Monts, August, 2015

LEO WAS GAZING at the horizon, between the sky and the ocean. He was looking at the surfers without really seeing them. Chloe and Sarah were splashing about in the waves on the beach. Paul was reading Michel Bussi's last book. The sky was picture-perfect blue, the sun was tanning nude skins, a slight breeze was drying drops of salty perspiration. Everything to have a great vacation with friends.

A few days before, Leo and Chloe had finished Noemie's diary, but the last page had been ripped out, and they remained dissatisfied with Sacha's digital confessions. Leo decided that it was probably better that way, that the deceased should have their secrets and tough luck for him if he didn't understand everything. He would remember his parents as determined to have a child, in spite of their difficulties, betrayals and lies, which most married couples probably had too.

They'd decided to put an end to their pseudo-investigations and take a week or two off for a vacation in Vendée. When Leo was little, he loved this part of France where he'd often gone on vacation with his parents.

Chloe thought about Paul and Sarah, their friends. Sarah studied with Chloe in the same university and they both had the summer off. Paul had his first job in a bank, and like Leo, was going to take a few weeks off too. That's how they'd all agreed to go to Saint-Jean-de-Monts the first two weeks in August where they'd rented a little cottage and split the cost, within walking distance of the beach.

So each day they went down to the seaside. Leo looked at Chloe lovingly: she was so beautiful in her little flowered bikini. Sarah wasn't bad either, he thought, looking over at Paul who was still immersed in *Black Water Lilies*.

"Hey Paul! Quit reading, quick," he yelled. "Sarah's being attacked by a shark! Run, you gotta try to save her!"

Paul, still zen, closed his paperback calmly, making sure the bookmark was on the right page.

"You're an idiot Leo. There aren't any sharks in Saint-Jean-de-Monts!"

"Okay, I give in. Is it a good book?"

I love Michel Bussi. He's got such original ideas. You ever read anything by him?"

"No, never heard of him. "But if you finish it, I'll try it."

"So let me read then instead of listening to your dumb jokes."

Paul went back to reading his whodunit and Leo laid down on his back, closed his eyes and basked in the warm summer sun.

He suddenly was aroused from his daydreaming by a shower of cold water. He jumped up. Chloe was wringing out her long blond hair above his chest.

"Just wait till I catch you!" he said, jumping up. She ran off. He ran after her. He quickly caught up with her, scooped her off her feet and rolled her around in the white sand. They burst out laughing and gave each other a big kiss. They were happy, they were in love, they'd forgotten everything else.

They spent the next several days carefree, relaxing, sightseeing, drinking wine and eating ice-cream cones. They also toured Noirmoutier Island, taking the *Passage du Gois*, this road that can only be used during low tide, and consequently only twice a day. Everyone had to wait in their cars until the ocean drew back, uncovering the cobblestones and asphalt with their ocean spray.

In the evening they played board games, had

barbecues or walked along the beach. A perfect vacation.

As their stay was drawing to an end though, Leo began to think about his parents' mysteries. One evening while all four of them were having a *Troussepinette*, the regional cocktail, Leo felt that he needed to talk about all this with his friends.

He summed up everything that had happened and everything they'd discovered: his parents' mortal accident, how he found his mom's diary, his dad's CD-ROM that someone had mysteriously put in the mailbox, Noemie's supposed infertility, that Maeva was his dad's mistress, as well as his suspicions that his mom also had an affair. His past that was turning out to be much more complex than he ever could have imagined

Then he admitted that he no longer wanted to delve into this ancient history, and that it would certainly be a better idea to ignore his family's mysterious history.

Would it be worse to know or not to?

"If I were you," Sarah said gently, "I don't think I'd be able not to try to find out more. Pandora's box and all that. I couldn't just close it like that. But curiosity is probably a very feminine flaw."

"But we're not you," added Paul. "It's your choice. Like the old saying goes: it's easy to give advice when you don't have to pay the price. Just ask yourself what's more important: wanting to know or fear of knowing? Curiosity or indifference?"

Leo thought this over.

"Maybe it's stupid, but my biggest question now after having found out all of this is what happened between the time that nothing was working out for them and the time I was born?"

"You mean that you're wondering whether it worked out naturally or your mom used medically assisted procreation?"

"I really have no idea about what I'm wondering about. Just that this doesn't seem to be normal, you know, that my parents had a skeleton in the closet."

"A secret then?" Sarah asked.

"Yeah, something like that."

They had another round of *Troussepinette*, religiously looking at its moiré reflections, then Sarah interrupted their ethylic silence.

"Leo, can I ask you a sort of delicate question?"

"Go ahead, we're all friends here."

"Okay. Here I go: did you ever think that you might have been adopted?"

That idea certainly shut all the friends up, and Leo only answered the question a few minutes later.

"You mean like my parents adopted me?"

"It's a possibility," Sarah continued.

That's something I never even thought about, but you're right, it's not impossible."

"Easy to find out," Sarah mused.

"How?"

"Did you ever see any pictures of your mother when she was pregnant?"

"You're right!" Chloe said. "I never saw any pictures where Noemie was pregnant. Strange, isn't it?"

Leo had no other choice than to silently agree, as he'd never seen any photos either, plus it was something that had never even seemed peculiar to him!

He thought back on their visit to his parents' house a few weeks ago and the photos on the wall. His parents when they got married, photos of him when he was a baby, then a little boy, then a teen and finally when he graduated. But nothing between when they got married and when he was born. A chronological hole in their lives.

So why weren't there any pictures of Noemie when she was pregnant? Or if there were, why weren't they up on the wall too? Where were they?

Leo couldn't stop thinking about this for the rest of their vacation. Now he couldn't wait to get back to Besancon to solve this mystery. His curiosity had again been roused. He couldn't wait to get back to his family's history.

When they got back home, Leo and Chloe rushed off to Noemie and Sacha's house, trying to find the answers to their new questions.

After a new but unsuccessful trip up to the attic, Chloe had the intuition that there might be some clues in Noemie's office. That's where she prepared her courses, corrected her papers, and maybe even wrote in her diary.

There was a typewriter and a few pencil holders as well as a ream of paper and a few magazines on top of her mahogany desk. Eight drawers on both sides of the chair, two of which were locked.

Leo went through the first six but didn't find anything.

"If she wanted to hide something, it must be in one of these two drawers," Chloe said.

"We have to find the key first."

"Where would you hide a key to your desk?"

"Anywhere I guess. In the office or someplace else."

"I'm sure she didn't hide it at the other end of the house, that wouldn't be very practical. Did you ever read Poe's story, *The Purloined Letter*? The people had looked all over and finally realized that the letter they'd been looking for was right in front of them!"

"You're right! The best way to hide something is to put it right in front of you. So, on the desk maybe?"

Leo went through the drawers once again, making sure the key wasn't attached to the bottom, the sides, or the top. No luck.

"The pencil holders!" Chloe shouted.

She took them and emptied them out on the desktop. And in the middle of the pens, pencils, erasers and scissors, there was a tiny bronze key. She handed it to Leo.

"This is for you, Sherlock!"

Leo put the key successively into the two drawers and rummaged around. Yet he couldn't rid himself from this feeling of shame, feeling he was violating his mother's sanctuary. Did he have the right to meddle in Noemie's locked up documents? Chloe realized he was upset.

"Honey, all we're looking for are some pictures! We don't care about the rest!"

Then he found a large envelope with

N+S= L written on it.

They'd hit the jackpot.

Leo opened it up and found a bunch of old faded photos in it.

He was astonished. Far from finding the answers to his questions, this discovery sparked a whole bunch of new questions.

Why hide the pictures of his mom when she was pregnant? Why dissimulate the very image of happiness?

What did this voluntary renunciation mean?

Now Leo really wanted to know more.

Chapter 32

February, 2015

THE TRUCK HAD JUST REACHED France coming in from Switzerland when the sun was rising over the snowy plains in Alsace.

Pippo was listening to the best of Eros Ramazzotti. An Italian listening to Eros could be seen as a cliche, but he loved this singer with his twangy voice, so different from the throaty voices other Italian singers had. Plus his tubes made him feel good, woke him up.

Pippo had stopped to sleep for a few hours on the last Swiss truck stop, the one in Pratteln. He preferred to shower and shave in Swiss facilities rather than in France, they were much cleaner.

He'd spent several minutes in the hot shower, rubbing his body, washing his hair. The hot water had eased the pain in his knee. Drops slid over the long scar on his kneecap that the doctors had done their best on.

When he was sitting in his truck, thinking about his shower, Pippo unconsciously rubbed his left knee. This wound was like a symbol of his failed life. The purple blistered scar with its permanent white spots on it was both a wound in his body and his heart.

He was still young when he exploded his knee. His whole life was in front of him. He even dreamed of glory and stardom. He could have become someone, had a good job, become a VIP, someone who they'd roll out the red carpet for. He would have traveled all over Europe and even the world… but not in a semi!

That was before. Before his busted knee.

Before this bitch who caused it, who was guilty. That lady he'd met, who he stayed with for a while, who he even had projects with. Who he could have associated with his prestige, had she been a bit more comprehensive, a bit less… exclusive! A young and good-looking guy like Pippo was not meant for only one woman, she should have understood that and accepted it, right? He would have given her money, showered her with jewels, purchased designer clothes for her, taken her to gala dinners. What else could she have wanted?

Had she just put her jealousy away in a cupboard, things would have been different.

And he wouldn't be here, driving down the highway from Basel to Mulhouse to Freiburg, with a load full of Pirelli tires. Instead of that he could have been dining with the Pirellis!

All that, plus everything else, that dark ten-year-old long parenthesis in his life, all that was Her fault!

Now it was payback time.

Pippo shifted gears. The semi blew a cloud of black smoke over the white Alsatian snow.

Part II

Chapter 33

Paris, May, 1989

THE INDIVIDUAL CROSSED the wooded square. Night had fallen on the capitol much earlier. Had he come across anyone, that person could have said that he'd seen a slim man, walking with determination towards some precise place.

It was true that the man seemed to be walking straight ahead, towards the many little pavilions that were in the institution: he seemed to be familiar with this place.

Leaves that had fallen from the birch and weeping willow trees crackled beneath his feet.

He neared Building C1, an old Haussmann-style building. Though the stones were old, to get in at night you needed to put a magnetic card into a lock, and he pulled it out of his dark grey coat.

The key box beeped sharply, the glass door slid open.

Inside, the only light came from the green panels indicating the emergency exits. At this time of night there were neither any visitors nor employees. It was logical and he must have known that as he didn't seem to care about being discreet. He however didn't turn on the lights right away and walked down the long hall, guided only by the greenish and spectral lighting from the ceiling.

He walked about thirty feet to another door, which had a digital code on it. Just as easy to get in as the front door. He quickly keyed it in as if he had mentally repeated this operation before coming, unless it was just something he was used to doing.

Had there been a guardian doing the rounds that night, would he have called out to him or just greeted him? His assertive attitude made you wonder.

This time the door didn't beep when opening, but just made a little click that the man waited for before turning the grey metal doorknob.

The room was semi-dark, light only came from a myriad of blue, red, green or orange buttons. A whole series of machines made the room look like a kitchen for municipalities. Huge refrigerators, freezers, cupboards, kitchen robots, yogurt makers and mixers were there making you think you were in a kitchen, except for the test tubes, Bunsen burners, containers for syringes or hair nets that were next to them.

The nocturnal visitor went directly to a container that he opened by lifting a windowed cover. Some vapor that seemed to be freezing immediately escaped from the container in a cloud surrounding his head, creating a halo and giving him a phantasmagorical look.

One after another he took the test tubes out and then put them back in. He did this at least ten times. Finally he looked closely at the eleventh, frowned, bringing it right up to his eyes as if he were looking for a tiny trace, something barely visible with the naked eye.

This was what he'd been looking for.

He hesitated, still holding it. He knew this wasn't right, he knew he was irresponsible, nearly criminal.

But he'd promised.

He felt like a god: all powerful.

Only one contradiction, one "entity" that could have dissuaded him from committing the irreparable: his own conscience.

He debated with it.

Then they agreed on a decision.

Chapter 34

Milan, October, 2015

LEO WAITED, sitting on a thermoformed plastic bench, looking at the conveyor belt where he was supposed to pick up his baggage. He didn't think he'd got the wrong one, as for the sixth time he reread the screen that said Alitalia 4912 - Orly. He was still wondering what, after a summer of doubt and reflection, finally made him want to go to Italy, a noisy country of voices that he'd heard for the first time, as there was a lively Italian family next to him, waiting like he was doing for their suitcases in Malpensa Airport.

Three months earlier, he'd been listening to his father's confessions on his laptop when the CD-ROM had frozen...

Chapter 35

Besançon, End of August 2015

WHEN HE GOT BACK from his vacation, Leo tried once again with his dad's CD-ROM. After having clicked several times and sworn once or twice, he tried to launch the video once again, but it froze at the same place. He'd right clicked on the scroll bar, hoping he'd be able to skip the defective sequence and hop to his father's confessions a bit farther on as now he was hooked.

Nothing worked though and Leo was ready to give up when he thought about his old laptop he'd put away in his bedroom closet. Did it still work? He doubted it.

He plugged it in and with a glimmer of hope, saw it light up. He put in the CD-ROM, and it immediately started reading it right at the beginning, the scene that had made him cry.

But it froze at the same place.

Now there was nothing to do, it was defective and that was it.

Leo would never know what else his father wanted to tell him.

He was so frustrated. Just like in all the Hollywood blockbusters, good characters, a thick plot and right when things were really getting interesting, nothing.

What would the outcome be ?

How did this passionate adventure end? Or had it actually ended or was Sacha still seeing his Italian mistress when the accident happened in 2015?

And why did he want to confess all this to his son?

Leo was sure he was missing the most important part. But how to find out? Faced with the tragic absence of the two main characters in this love triangle, would he be able to find the third one? Was this Maeva lady still alive? Where? How could he find her? A first name, a city, a foreign airline: three slim clues for someone who was neither Hercule Poirot nor Columbo.

Maybe one day his father had talked to one of his close friends or family members. And as he had not been brave enough to confess his affair to his son, maybe it had been something he'd spoken about to his best friend?

LEO CALLED LOIC, his father's childhood friend, one who he still saw when he was an adult. A sincere friend, who'd been there for Leo when he needed him.

"Loic, I have to see you. You have to tell me about my dad."

"I'm home, come whenever you want."

Loic was seated across from his best friend's son, each one in the comfortable armchairs in his restaurant.

Two half-full cups of coffee on the table.

"You know, you can always count on me, Leo," Loic said for the third time. "For anything!"

"Great then," said Leo, not really knowing how to ask him that burning question. "Did you know my dad was having an affair?"

Loic remained silent, then sighed and picked up his cup of coffee, took a few sips and squinted from the hot steam it gave off. He put his cup back down finally.

"You should look towards the future rather than living in the past. It's never a good idea to wake up the dead. I'm sorry to be so blunt here Leo, but I think your parents deserve to rest in peace, like everyone else who needs to find peace within themselves."

"But did he tell you he was having an affair?"

"Your father loved your mother," Loic said, not

answering the question. "That I can guarantee you. You can't even imagine how he described her to me when they first met at the university. It was love at first sight for them and after thirty years, I'm sure they still loved each other. They were an intensely close couple. It was crazy to see them after so many years walking together in the streets, stopping to kiss each other tenderly."

Loic's voice choked up while thinking back on their youth together. Looking down at his cup, running a hand through his hair, he seemed to be lost, aware of the emptiness now surrounding them. Interminable seconds went by before he could speak again.

"When you were born, that was the happiest moment in their lives. They wanted you so much! Your dad did tell me about how hard it was for them to conceive. Then you finally arrived, and you were the cement binding them together, the living symbol of the fusional love they had for each other!"

"Loic, I know all that. I know that my dad really loved my mom. But I also know that he loved another woman."

"What on earth makes you think that?"

"I didn't have to look too far. My dad admitted it. Well, not directly, when he was still alive. I realize you're trying to protect me, I know that you think back on my parents like they could do no wrong, like they were an ideal couple! But my dad admitted this himself: '*everything's not black or white, but different shades of grey.*' And I'm trying to make sense of this shade of grey, with your help, if possible. How about another cup of coffee?"

"I'd personally prefer a whisky, that would loosen up my tongue."

"I'll have one too then!"

Loic filled two glasses and Leo continued.

"My dad left me - and I still don't know how I got it - a testimonial on a CD-ROM. You know how much he loved IT! All the stuff you just told me, stuff I didn't know before, he told me all that too. And I'm happy to say that what he said is what we all saw. So anyway, I'm asking you for help here because that damn CD crashed right when he was telling me about someone called Maeva, an Italian that he went out with before I was born. You know anything about that?"

Loic took a sip of his eighteen-year-old Chivas Regal, pursed his lips and let out a long breath before starting.

"I think she was a flight attendant."

"Right! I was sure he told you about her, you were his best friend! So what else do you know?"

"Not much, to tell the truth. Of course, he'd told me about her, like you talk to your friends when you're having a glass of Picon beer at the local bar. He told me how audacious he was when he was flying to Milan. What a guy, Sacha! Something I never would have done! And he did tell me what happened between them, though he loved your mother. He said he was spellbound by her Italian charm."

"Did he show you a picture of her?"

"Never. But I'm sure she must have been something else to make him fall for her like that. At least an Italian Madonna to make him forget your mother's dazzling beauty for a weekend."

"Just a weekend? Or did that last?"

"They might have seen each other again. They would have been able to as his boss got a whole bunch of other contracts in Milan."

"Did he go there often?"

"For a couple of years, he had to go there quite often, each time for a week. He'd leave Monday morning and come back Friday in the evening. But he just told me about the first time. After that, I don't know if he went back to Milan just for work or if he saw her again. A one-night-stand or a longer affair? *That is the question!*"

"You just know her first name?"

"Her first name, the city where they met, her job, nothing more than you do."

"I'm sure there was really something between them. He wouldn't have told me about a simple one-night-stand. To err is human and accidents happen. Lots of couples go through that. In a life of twenty-five or thirty years as a couple, who can say they were never tempted to have an adventure, or never hoped for one? Just one night? Passion of someone else, someone new. So, had this been the case, my dad wouldn't have... wouldn't have wanted to hurt me with something like this. There was something else going on here and I want to know what!"

You're inventing things Leo!"

"Stop it! Please. Help me track down this Maeva who seems to have played a key role in my father's life."

Loic had taken the last sip of whisky in his glass.

"Okay. I'll help you because you won't give up. But I already told you everything I know. Do you even know if she's still alive? If she still lives in Italy? Or in France maybe? We don't have any good clues here, like a last name, an address, a phone number or an email account. Something even Columbo couldn't solve!"

"Good Lord! Why didn't I think of that earlier?"

"Think of what?"

"His BlackBerry! It's not like I want to be scouring around in a dead person's stuff, but I'm sure I could find something there. My dad had an accident unfortunately. And if he had stuff he'd wanted to hide, he didn't have the time to delete it."

"You think you can find some emails? Maybe her phone number?"

"I sure hope so. All the personal belongings he had with him the day of the accident are still in the trunk of the car."

They quickly went out and came back with the box that the cops had given him and where they'd put all the various objects and personnel documents they'd found in the car and in the victim's pockets.

Almost embarrassed by what he was doing and sad to have to be doing it, Leo took out the phone that his dad used for work.

Of course the battery was dead.

"Wait a sec, I've got an old phone charger someplace," said Leo. He found it in his office with a bunch of other old cables and connected it to the phone.

The screen lit up, displaying its traditional message:

"*Enter your PIN code,*" shit!

What could it be?

How many numbers? Certainly four, like most PINs.

Leo was disheartened by the immensity of the probable PIN codes to be discovered without any clues.

He keyed in "0000," which was the default code of all phones, without believing for a single moment that his father wouldn't have changed it the first time he used it.

"*Invalid PIN code.*"

"Okay. What I'd figured."

"Why don't you try a date?" suggested Loic. "Their wedding, when they first met?"

"Sure, but which one? His, mine, my mom's? Or even Maeva's, why not?

"It's hard to tell, that's for sure. Plus you've only got two more tries before the SIM card automatically blocks. So you'd better think this over and pray for "*la Buona Fortuna*! What's your PIN code?"

"My birthday. What about you?"

"Same thing."

Loic poured them both a double dose of whisky to help them think and Leo had an idea.

"I'm going to try their wedding date."

He keyed in the four numbers and pressed "Enter" but had that same old message, "*Error PIN code*," followed by another one that was just as stressful, "*Last try*." He felt like giving up, not wanting to try for the last time, wanting to forget about Maeva, their affair, cheating, following Loic's advice to let time heal those old wounds of existence.

Both Loic and he finished their glasses.

"Come on, we've got one try left," said Loic. "I've got an idea here, I don't know what it's worth, but we can give it a try. When you think about everything you know about your dad, what was the most important thing for him?"

"Mom?"

"We already tried their wedding date: it didn't work. And for your mom?"

"Me. So you think his code is my birthday?"

"I'd sure bet ten bucks on it! If it hadn't been so old hat, they would have called you 'Desired.'"

Leo grabbed the BlackBerry and put in the day and month of his birth.

Four stars on the screen and then an orange light on its facade. The date and time came on, the five bars of satellite reception, the logo of the service supplier and then the wallpaper...

A photo of Leo when he was little.

Tears suddenly welled up in his eyes faced with this secret proof of how much his father loved him, even having his picture on his professional phone.

"Jesus, we're in!

All we have to do now is look through his address book for her contact details. Find a phone number, an address, an email.

I won't be able to do this. Loic, can you do it?" said Leo, handing the phone to him.

A few minutes and another whisky later, those cyber investigators had only found one email that could correspond to their research, but they were sure it was the right one:

mae.dannunzio@gmail.com

Chapter 36

Milan, October, 2015

LEO PICKED up his bag from the baggage claim belt. He threw it over his shoulder and went out to the taxi rank in front of Milan Malpensa Airport.

"Hilton Hotel," he told the chauffeur.

He took advantage of the trip to call Chloe, say he'd arrived and that he was both excited and worried about this trip and that he loved her and he knew that he'd be able to count on her whatever happened here.

And while looking at the Milan suburbs through the taxi windows, Leo thought back on last week, which was why he'd decided to go to Italy.

The email that he'd sent was what had triggered this trip to the past.

Chapter 37

Besançon, August 31, 2015

FROM: *Leo Terebus leothefirst@gmail.com*
To:mae.dannunzio@gmail.com
Object: My father, Sacha Terebus
Hello,
First of all, I'd like to apologize if you are not the right person for this message.
And I'm also sorry that I can't write to you in Italian.
Please allow me to introduce myself: my name is Leo, but if you're the person I think you are, you must know that I exist.
So I'm Sacha's son and he confessed that he met you over twenty-five years ago when he was in Milan for business.
Today I'm still grieving for him (and for my mother, Noemie). But before he passed away, he'd left me his confessions, in which you seem to have played a key role.

. . .

I UNFORTUNATELY WAS NOT *able to access the totality of his testimonial and I still have several questions that remain unanswered.*

I'm sure that you have some answers, and this is why I decided to write to you.

If you want to, if you're brave enough or if you simply want to pay tribute to the memory of this man who fell madly in love with you, you can answer this email or call me at....

I'm looking forward to hearing from you.

Best regards,

Leo Terebus.

Leo clicked on "Send" and made sure that he message had been sent. He'd not even wondered up till now if the email address he'd seen was still valid. He quickly went into his "Messages sent" file, fearing that he'd see the "Undeliverable mail" or "Unknown Address "messages in it.

After half an hour though, nothing had come back. His message had been sent and had surely arrived.

Would someone read it? Would it really be Maeva at this address? Would she respond?

⁓

HE HAD to wait about two weeks before he had an answer.

. . .

FROM: MAEVA D'ANNUNZIO « MAE.DANNUNZIO@GMAIL.COM»

To:leothefirst@gmail.com
Object: Re: My father, Sacha Terebus
Buona sera, Leo!
Yes, I'm that Maeva that your father told you about.
I still live in Milan and I've never forgotten Sacha, I want you to know this.
But I'm not brave enough to answer your many questions. At least not by email.
On the other hand, I really would like you to come, if possible of course, and see me in Milan so we can both talk.
The earlier the better.
There are daily flights from Paris, Lyon, or Geneva to Milan Malpensa with Alitalia (www.alitalia.it).
Tell me which flight would be the best and I'll transfer the tickets to you.
Don't worry about accommodations, I'll take care of everything!
I'm looking forward to hearing from you.
Maeva.

Both excited and apprehensive, Leo had thus followed Maeva's instructions. She had sent him the plane tickets as well as a voucher for a room at the Hilton in the center of Milan. That's how, in October, he first set foot in Italy where he hoped he'd be finding answers to the many questions he had after hearing his father's unfinished confessions.

Chapter 38

Milan, October, 2015

LEO TEREBUS WAS BARE CHESTED, standing in front of the mirror in the bathroom in the hotel. He still had shaving cream on his face and was holding his razor, unable to move. He suddenly realized what upset him last night, when he spent the evening with this person he didn't know. The solution jumped right out at him. He couldn't deny it. Everything suddenly was crystal-clear, or he could also have said, obvious, like the nose in the middle of his face.

∽

LEO WAS the first to arrive in the bar in the center of Milan where they'd agreed to meet. He looked at the door apprehensively, hesitating between curiosity, fear and relief to finally be able to shed light on the troubled past of his parents.

People came in, others went out, a great Mediterranean atmosphere filled the bar with laughter, people shouting and these typical Italian gestures making you think that these people talked with their hands and their words were only there to illustrate what they thought.

Would he recognize her amongst the crowd of anonymous customers? He visualized how he thought she'd look, especially as he'd listened one more time to that old CD-ROM where his father described her with so much passion. Plus, she'd told him in her last email that she'd be wearing a light, yellow dress and a straw hat, so he wouldn't be able to miss her.

And then he saw her come in...

No doubt. It was HER. Of course, the hat and dress helped, but there was something else. Something he couldn't put his finger on, but that could only be her, he was sure.

She walked right up to him. He got up and extended his hand. She held onto it with her fingertips, smiling and then said in her singsong voice:

"Datemi un baccio! Give me a kiss!"

Feeling her cheeks, the scent of her perfume! Leo felt an undefinable trouble. In just a few seconds he'd understood why his father had fallen head over heels in love with this woman! He himself, right now and despite their difference in age - nearly thirty years which had left no traces on her - he himself felt her attraction. His father's blood ran through his veins, so he wasn't astonished that it also inundated his heart with the same hot Italian fire.

"*Caro mio, sirvami un Biancho per favore,*" she said to the waiter when she sat down.

She started up the conversation, as Leo hadn't yet opened his mouth.

"What do you think of Milan?"

"Enchanting!"

"Is the hotel alright?"

"Oh! Yes, thank you. But you needn't have reserved a hotel that's so…"

"Expensive?"

"I was going to say chic."

"Hey. Don't worry about that. My employer, Alitalia, has a partnership with the Hilton group. I've got pretty good prices everywhere! And even more so in Milan."

"Anyway, thanks for having agreed to meet me, especially in these circumstances."

Leo could feel that Maeva was uncomfortable.

"Leo, I did love your father. I'm very sorry for your loss. And for your mother too. I'd like you to know that I sincerely share your pain."

"That's nice of you."

"No, it's sincere. I know I don't play the good role in this story. I was your father's mistress. But I do hope that I didn't hurt your mother. And I hope she never found out about us... never! Had she found out, what would she have done?"

"Probably like most wives who find out their husband has been cheating on them: served him divorce papers. Or maybe not, knowing her, she would have fought like a lion to keep my father next to her!"

"And I would have liked that to have been the case, for all three of you!"

Heavy thoughts were going through their heads while they were having their cocktails. Then Leo asked a question that was important for him.

"How long were you two together?"

"When I met Sacha, I'd just gotten out of a complicated relationship, one that wasn't pleasant at all. I promised myself that I'd never fall in love with another man, I didn't want to belong to anyone, I wanted to live my own life, at my own rhythm, with no constraints. And then your father entered my life like a meteorite falling onto the earth: at lightning speed and burning! He wanted to see me again, once, twice, three times. And each time he went back to France, I surprised myself by wanting him to come back to Milan again on business. It was like a habit for both of us. Something that suited both of us perfectly. We were passionately together for a few days, without ever promising anything at all. And I certainly wasn't going to ask my lover to get divorced! I knew he was happy at home and so was I."

"Have you ever been married?"

"Never! Marriage wasn't for me."

"Do you have any children?"

"Ah! Children... My only regret. It's too late now though."

She laughed nervously. A quick and sharp laugh, with a shade of contained sadness in it.

"You're still *una bella donna*," said Leo. "The Italian sun must be a true fountain of youth."

"You're sweet Leo, but you never saw me when I wake up!"

"How long did your adventure with my dad last?" Leo asked once again.

"The last time I saw Sacha was six months ago. So you can see it was far from a one-night-stand, something that lasted a whole lifetime!"

"Wow! How could my father have had a double life for almost thirty years?"

"Maybe because it was a double passion. Do you believe in stuff like that Leo?"

"I think it's possible, at least I mean that it certainly worked for my father. Would you like another glass? Talking so much dries your tongue out!"

"With pleasure! Mario, *un'altro giro*!"

"Now that I think about it, you must have known that Sacha had a son?"

"*Mamma mia*! Of course! Your father was so overjoyed! No way could I have not known!"

"But when they finally succeeded in having a child, that didn't make him want to break up with you?"

"We talked about it a couple of times, but each time he said that he needed this double anchor. But our relationship became one of just two friends. Very good friends, powerfully linked to each other, see?"

"I guess I can imagine that," agreed Leo, successively drowning in his glass of Martini and in Maeva's eyes. "Did you always meet here in Milan?

"Most of the time. Far from home, Sacha didn't feel as guilty. Even though as a flight attendant, I was often in Paris or Lyon. We could have seen each other there, but he was reluctant, something I understand. But we did see each other in France a couple of times, just for a change of scenery!"

"And I can't believe that my mom never found out about this! And I didn't either! I mean like when I was a kid, I understand, but when I grew older and became an adult, I could have had some doubts, wondered why he was gone, understood what wasn't being said, or maybe surprised at some mistakes he made... Nothing though! Not a thing! Plus I always felt, and I'm sure it was true, that I was a part of a close family, surrounded by two parents who loved me and who loved each other."

"That was the case, I confirm it. Listen Leo, I want to tell you something that I feel is important."

"I'm listening, Maeva. That's sort of like why I'm here! To find out more about this. Understand this facet of my father, my parents, something that I never even suspected before the accident."

Leo could feel that Maeva was troubled. He realized that words were having trouble coming out of her luscious lips.

"It's getting stuffy here in the bar. How about going outside?"

"Fine with me! You're the guide."

Maeva paid for the drinks and they walked down the streets toward the river banks. While they walked, until they arrived at the banks of the *Naviglio Grande*, silences followed small talk about how warm it was, how beautiful the buildings were, how nice it was just to walk without having to be on time somewhere. Maeva took Leo by the arm.

"I didn't tell you everything about when I was in France. It's true, I didn't come there often, I only stayed for a stopover or just a weekend. But one day, Sacha asked me if I wanted to meet you. I hesitated for a while about being introduced to his son. But he finally convinced me. He told me he was happy to introduce me to his son he was so proud of! I'm sure you don't remember; you were really young then."

"We already met?"

"Briefly, but yes. Sacha asked me to go to

Micaud Park in Besancon, a little park right on the Doubs River, across from Mercure Hotel where I was staying. He told me to wait on one of the benches near the newsstand, about four-thirty when schools got out. I remember that the school was near there, rue d'Helvétie, I think."

"That's right. I was in pre-school there."

"You must have been three or four. I saw you coming, hand in hand, to meet me. I nearly ran away."

"How come?"

"Just because it was so weird, you know, meeting my lover's child, right there, right next to your school, in your everyday lives. I suddenly felt so... foreign I guess, right then, like I didn't fit into your beautiful family."

"Did you stay though?"

"Yes, I did. Sacha introduced you to me as '*someone who worked with Daddy.*' He told you '*Say hello to the lady, her name is Maeva, isn't that a nice name?*' I remember that as if it were yesterday, but now here you are, holding me by the arm, and I just say to myself that it's incredible how time flies. I bent down to give you a kiss on the cheek and you said: '*Hello, Miss Maeva.*' You were so cute! After that, the three of us walked in the park, you and Sacha were still holding hands and I was walking next to you."

"Just like a real family, right?"

"Just like a real family. *Si vero*, we could have been," Maeva sighed.

"I must have been really little because I don't remember that at all. I don't think kids remember anything before they're at least three. But there must have been something."

"Really? What?"

"Well, when you walked into the bar, without the shadow of a doubt I immediately knew that you were the one I was waiting for. Like for some unclear reason, I recognized you."

"Maybe there was some obscure memory of my face hidden inside your brain, in one of the compartments of your childhood, one that was locked when you became an adult. And maybe it opened when I walked into the bar!"

"Do you believe in stuff like that? I mean, stuff hidden in your subconsciousness?"

"I think the human brain and memory are more complicated than we could ever imagine. Our unconscious life is a thousand times richer than our conscious life."

"Come on," Leo said, laughing. "Let's not have such an intellectual discussion here for such a nice night out in Milan!"

"You're right young man: in Milan we laugh, we don't cogitate!"

They both laughed and then silently both thought over this last sentence. Leo finally interrupted their meditations.

"And I never saw you since?"

"No, never. You never saw me, but I often saw you!"

"Like you were spying on me?"

"Not at all. Sacha always showed me pictures of you. He was so overjoyed to see you growing up, you, his only son, the one they'd been waiting for so long to have, that he couldn't help but talking about you each time we met. *'And look how big he's getting,'* and *'You know he has really good grades in class,'* or *'He just turned ten,'* and *'Look, now he's a teenager, with those eyes the girls are going to be crazy about him!'* He couldn't shut up about you, a real chatterbox, worse than a girl!"

"And all that stuff about his happy family, that didn't bother you?"

"No, on the contrary!"

"Really?"

"Of course. I loved knowing what was going on. I already said: things were always very clear between Sacha and me. He had his perfect family life, I was his hidden mistress, and I never asked him for anything else than love, as a family life wasn't my thing. I loved seeing him so happy!"

"And were you happy too?"

"I think so. I was happy to make him happy, happy by proxy maybe."

"Just goes to say that people find happiness wherever they can!" concluded Leo.

Chapter 39

Milan, Hilton Hotel, October, 2015

LEO WAS STILL HOLDING his razor. He was finding it hard to emerge from his thoughts where he kept on going through the conversation he'd had last night with Maeva, his father's mistress. The shaving cream on his cheeks was starting to drip while his own reflection kept on jumping out at him, especially his nose... that nose that seemed to be wanting to tell him something! He was submerged by a huge doubt, nearly sure of something that had come from someplace, and that he wasn't sure he believed! Would that have been possible? Or was he just inventing a very improbable scenario here?

He had to make sure. He decided his shave was good enough and rinsed off his cheeks with warm water and ran to pick up his phone. While he was looking for the number in his contacts, someone knocked at the door.

"*Signor!* A letter for you. Someone put it at the reception desk. *Prego.*"

Leo picked up the envelope, opened it while continuing to look for the phone number with his other hand.

While his left thumb was getting ready to press "Call," to join Maeva, his right hand opened the envelope that had a simple and brief sentence.

Leo, if you want to know who you are and where you come from, join me at the hotel bar. Maeva.

∞

LEO SAW Maeva sitting in an angle of the lobby, in front of a glass of champagne with a black olive in it. He joined her, looking right at her. She herself seemed mummified. He looked right into her face that now seemed familiar to him. Neither of them seemed to be able to break that wall of silence weighing them down, that mystery that Leo believed he had solved and that made him question her.

"How did that happen?"

A huge question, one that quickly generated a whole bunch of others in his head and that overturned everything he'd discovered in the past horrible weeks after his parents died.

"I can explain everything. Sit down here, next to

me." Leo found her tone of voice much more natural than the day before. She seemed to realize this.

"I can't talk to you as if I just met you as a stranger, is that okay? You're so young."

"That's fine. But please don't take any offense if the opposite is still hard for me."

"That's understandable. You just met me, you came to Milan thinking you'd meet your father's mistress - which is true - and now in just a few hours you're starting to notice a lot of other more... more incredible things. So sure, I can understand that you're not comfortable with me. Even though I hope that what I'll tell you will bring back a bit of happiness that you lost when your parents disappeared."

"Since yesterday, your face kept haunting me, all I could see was your eyes, your mouth, your nose. Then this morning when I was shaving..."

"You must have said to yourself: '*I must be dreaming!*' But it's not a dream Leo. Even though it seems like one. The background is hazy, time is elastic, imprecise, the characters are intertwined in your head I'd imagine? We're going to try to unravel all of that together, calmly, step by step."

"Okay. Where are we going to start?" asked Leo, holding his head in his hands and punctuating the sentence with a sigh.

"I'd like to go back to the very beginnings of this, if it's alright with you. Let me tell you about the discussion I had with your dad when he was here once. That night he was despondent, completely depressed by all the failures that he and your mom had had since they'd been trying to conceive. That was all he could think about, and he said..."

Chapter 40

Milan, December, 1988

... WHEN STRAIGHTENING up against the headboard:

"I can't stand it anymore, *Cara mia*! I'm going crazy. What on earth did I do to the good Lord to deserve this?"

"Because you're a believer now?"

"Just a French expression. Maybe I should believe in God, that could help us! A little helping hand from fate, and there you go! The miracle of Conception! Bullshit! How can people still believe in the Immaculate Conception that the Holy Ghost breathed into Mary when even the most famous doctors can't even give me the child I want so badly?"

"That's blasphemous dear, don't forget that

you're in Italy, not so far from the Vatican! Come here, I'll console you."

"I don't want to be consoled; I want a kid!" Sacha nearly shouted this, in a heartfelt cry.

"Hey there. Just a minute. I don't have to take crap like this. If you want to talk, I'm here, if not, *basta*."

Sacha calmed down.

"I'm sorry. Can you understand though that I'm going nuts? Sometimes I think I'll just give up: leave my sterile wife, start over again someplace else with someone else and have a real family! Not just a couple."

"What about adoption? There are so many unhappy little orphans in the world that would love to be a part of a family, they'd love to be loved by a happy couple. And I know that you and your wife are made for one another. So why spoil all that?"

"What if you gave me that child?"

The sentence hit her just like a whip, no one said anything then Maeva spoke up.

"Sacha, I already told you, I've kissed all that goodbye. Being your mistress, an occasional fuck, my freedom, that's all I want. So a husband and a kid fulltime, no thanks!"

"Why? That's what most women want, don't they?"

"I'm not most women! I'm me, I've got my own personal history and my own desires for the future. And I don't want to be tied down."

"What made you be so independent? You never told me about your past, Maeva. Your parents got divorced and you became so bitter that you never wanted to get married? Your father beat you or your mother? What could have broken the strongest human desire in you: giving life?"

"Dr. Sacha, can I lie down on your couch? Since when did you become a shrink? Leave me alone with your questions!"

Sacha snuggled up against Maeva.

"*Cara mia, bellissima*, I've been listening to you and watching you for several months now, ever since we've been together and I know that something happened. I'd like to know what. I'm ready to listen all night long if that's what it takes."

He kissed her earlobe.

"Tell me about your past."

"*Va bene!* The night is still young... Let me start off by saying that I never had any problems with my parents! They loved each other, took good care of us, me and my sisters, Giuliana and Vittoria, maybe I already told you about them. They still live together in their little home in Apulia, I stop by when I can, between two flights, and I send them postcards from each new port of call! See, a perfect family life."

"So maybe things went wrong when you were a teen? A pimple-faced kid maybe? That's why now, as you're so beautiful, you flit from man to man, never staying. A lovely butterfly that flies from flower to flower and drinks in nectar as it goes?"

"Wrong again, *Dottore*! When I was fifteen my skin was perfect. Girls were jealous of me in my village, and guys were happy!"

"So you were... precautious then."

"It's true, I loved men at an early stage. I started when I was young and I had a good collection. But I'm not going to describe my hunting bag to you, not tonight nor ever! So please stop interrupting me and you'll quickly understand why I can't have a child for you."

"Mum's the word my adorable Italian."

Maeva closed her eyes and took a deep breath before starting what seemed to be a confession she'd hidden deep in her heart. While speaking, her eyes remained closed.

"*WHEN I WAS EIGHTEEN, I met a man I fell madly in love with. He was twenty and he played in the reserve team for Milan AC. He was handsome, his future was cut out for him in soccer, in one of the best clubs in the world, and all the girls, like me, were in love with him and came to watch him train. And out of all these soccer groupies, I was the one he chose. I wasn't the most beautiful nor the most exciting one. We met in a nightclub where he and his teammates came to celebrate their victory. We saw each other more and more often, after the games, and then as we got on well together, we spent even more time together. He made a very good living and was housed free of charge in a little villa in the good suburbs of Milan and I joined him there each time my schedule let me. It wasn't always easy, both of us traveled so much, him with his games and me with my flights all over Europe.*

After two years together we decided to have a child and I got pregnant right away. In spite of our jobs, we wanted to have kids, you were right about this Sacha: that was how I saw my life then, a conformist, ticking all the boxes.

Then things started going downhill. Oh! Not because I was pregnant, everything was fine there. But because of his job. Filippo kept on going out a lot with his teammates. After each game, they'd party in a discotheque, whether they won or they lost: any excuse was a good one. But I was too tired to go with them. So I trusted him. Had I only known... With success and all the money he had, he started to drink, plus he started to smoke dope. Then soft drugs turned into hard ones, he started shooting up.

He still had flocks of girls surrounding him. You know, even when they're married, soccer players have a lot of temptation. I knew he was cheating on me.

We fought about this. I couldn't stand his behavior anymore, especially when he wasn't even hiding the fact!

And then one day my flight was canceled because of a strike and I came home much earlier than expected, without telling him, I wanted to surprise him! Talk about a surprise. He was with one of his bimbos and fucking her in the shower. That pig! I insulted them, I threw everything available at them: shampoo, razors, toothbrushes... And then the blond hit the road trying to cover her ass with one of Filippo's towels and he stayed in the shower like an idiot, eyes glazed over and his prick still erect from his interrupted fuck! Plus I could tell right away that he was as drunk as a skunk or maybe high or probably both, seeing the way he looked. I jumped on him and slammed my hand into his filthy cock. He yelled out holding his crotch. 'You bitch' he shouted at me - he didn't realize he was the one at fault here and then he hit me several times. I tried to run, calling for help, but I slipped on the wet tiles because of all the water his slut spilled when she ran off. I tried to protect my stomach by falling on my hands, but I sprained a wrist.

Had that been all, maybe I would have raised my kid alone and forgotten this guy.

But being half drunk and stoned, he didn't see things that way that night. I don't know if it's a masculine primary reflex, but when I slapped his dick - now a limp one - it must have driven him crazy and he literally took it out on me.

I was still on the floor and he kicked me repeatedly while yelling at me. I instinctively tried to protect my stomach by rolling up in a ball and hiding my head in my arms.

But that wasn't enough. He was out of control, and I think that was what did it, the man who I'd fallen in love with, the man with whom I'd made this baby, it wasn't Filippo who, standing above me, kept on kicking me..."

MAEVA HAD SLID down in the bed, her eyes still closed, in that very position she was describing to Sacha. Tears were pouring down on her cheeks and she was nearly suffocating.

"My beautiful Maeva, I'm here, calm down, all

of that happened a long time ago," said Sacha, trying to control her and holding her in his arms more tightly than an armor.

∽

MILAN, **Hilton Hotel, October, 2015**

LEO COULD FEEL the sadness and wrath in Maeva's voice when she told him about this traumatic experience that had taken place when she was young.

Like she had experienced the same pain for the third time. The first time was physical, with Filippo; the second, which was perhaps the hardest for her, was when she was in bed with Sacha, and the third was to explain to him why she'd chosen this life.

"You lost your baby?" asked Leo, to resume the dialog.

"Yes, I did. The fetus died *in utero* and I had to go to the ER to expel it. My sister Vittoria took me. Filippo was dead to the world, wallowing like the pig he was on the couch where he'd sat down after having left me like a rag on the wet tiles in the bathroom."

"What ever happened to him? Is he still a soccer player?"

"I don't think so. In fact, I'm sure he isn't. That night, while he was beating me, to try to defend myself, I grabbed his foot. He slipped on the wet tiles and fell down screaming. He was holding his knee that had slammed into the angle on the bathtub. I found out later that he had to have several operations, that his cruciate ligaments had been hit and that his rotula was pulverized. His career was finished, all his dreams of glory and fame were over. Plus I never saw his name again in the 90s in the Milan AC players. At the best, maybe he coaches a team of juniors!"

"He must have cursed you for the rest of his life then. But he deserved what he got. Plus you gave up wanting to have a family… After something like that, it must be terribly hard to recover."

"It was so awful, you know. We broke up, I even wanted to sue him, but decided not to. It just would have been like rubbing salt into my wound, which was so deep. But after that I swore to myself that I would never trust a man again, whoever he was. Get pregnant again, carry the promise of a new life, then fearing for nine months that everything could end… I even considered getting my tubes tied."

"It must have been awful," Leo agreed. But I don't understand how what you went through then and my questions about who I am are linked together. What has that got to do with me?"

"Leo, you're right in the heart of this story! Or maybe should I say at the end of the logical chain of reasoning. Do you think you're ready to hear the rest?"

"That's why I came. When I listened to your message while I was shaving this morning, I thought I'd understood some things, some truths that overturned the natural order of my family. And now you want me to understand stuff that seems to jeopardize what I thought I'd understood. Now I don't know what to think anymore."

"Because you don't know most of it. Let me tell you the rest."

Chapter 41

Paris, January, 1989

NOEMIE AND SACHA were in the waiting room of the specialist in gynecological genetics that Sacha had selected from the list that Dr. Lepic had given them. He was apparently one of the best, and he even gave conferences and spoke at congresses all around the world.

They'd thought about it for a long time and had finally decided to consult. Sacha had been the most tenacious one here and Noemie had followed him without much hope. She'd thought that rather than doing nothing, they had nothing to lose by trying. But she wasn't ready to do just anything, she didn't want to be a guinea pig for science. But her love for Sacha made her agree.

Now they were anxious to see this famous and reputable doctor.

His secretary opened the door of the waiting room.

"Mr. and Mrs. Terebus? Professor Siethbüller can see you now, just follow me," she said, pointing to two rattan armchairs.

They went into a large room with furniture made from the finest wood. The walls were full of shelves overflowing with medical encyclopedias and little African statuettes. The desk in front of them seemed to be made from lacquered walnut and was tidy, with only a manila file with their name on it on top of it.

The room was huge with high ceilings. It had two doors: the first one where they'd entered and the second one, on the right, where a tall and handsome man with salt and pepper colored hair came in.

"I'm pleased to meet you, Mr. and Mrs. Terebus. I hope I can help you," said Professor Siethbüller, holding out his hand.

"Thanks for taking our case, Professor," said Sacha.

"Hello," said Noemie, with a friendly smile.

The doctor sat down in a huge leather armchair and opened the couple's file.

"My colleague, Dr. Lepic, sent me your entire file. I've already gone through your exams. As she told you, you're one of the six percent of patients who really doesn't have a cause for their infertility, at least not in the current state of our medical knowledge."

"That's true, Dr. Lepic already told us the same thing," said Noemie.

"I don't want you to be frightened here," said Dr. Siethbüller, trying to reassure her. "That's why she sent you to me. I'm not a 'miracle-maker' but my work consists in trying to find the root cause of your infertility, and it's generally a genetic one. So then I try to find the best adapted solution to your case. To do this I've got cutting-edge equipment, a qualified and motivated team plus I use the latest and internationally recognized techniques. But I can't do anything without you!"

"Meaning?" asked Sacha, astonished.

"To start off with, you'll be the ones deciding whether or not to take a whole new bunch of tests, but I can reassure you, they're not medically invasive ones."

"Invasive?" exclaimed Noemie.

"Oh sorry for the medical talk and don't hesitate to interrupt me whenever I start using too many doctor's formulas. I just meant that the tests are not physically difficult ones. On the other hand, the results obtained from them could be hard to hear and accept. You have to be prepared for this."

"But how?" Noemie continued.

"By talking it over. Between you two and then with me. For us, these are expensive tests. And for you, the costs must be proportional to your degree of motivation to conceive, with medical assistance, because in your case this is what we're now looking at. Now we have to see how much medical assistance is actually required. And this is what the tests will tell us."

"If we came here," Sacha added, "it's because both of us want to know what the problem is and then be able to find a solution to it, Professor."

Professor Jacques Siethbüller nodded his head.

"That's what I think too. I called Dr. Lepic and she reassured me about this. I also saw when I looked at the dates, that your decision had the time to mature in your heads and certainly also in your hearts. With experience, I can also read this in your eyes."

"Are you going to be able to help us Professor?" asked Sacha.

"I'll do everything I can! Let me talk you through these tests. Here these are genetic ones. I was trained as a gynecologist but then I specialized in genetics, as I quickly understood that in the future, this discipline would become very important. Just look at how the Telethon has democratized research in genetics. Did you ever watch their show?"

They both nodded.

"So you've already heard words like chromosomal sequencing, karyotype, DNA, etc. That's what we'll be working with for you. I have to analyze this for both of you. The results I obtain will allow me to give you a very detailed and definitive diagnostic."

"How do you get all of that?" asked Noemie.

"It's easy for you: just by doing your bloodwork! See, it's not hard. But the blood we take will have to undergo a lot of tests in our equipment!"

"Perfect. When do we start?" Sacha asked.

"You can get this done today or tomorrow here in our lab. My secretary will give you an appointment. Any other questions?"

Noemie and Sacha must have had lots of other questions but didn't say a thing. They were holding hands, once again full of hope. Professor Siethbüller concluded his appointment.

"I'm sure you'll have more questions when we get the results. It'll take a good ten days and we'll see each other again then. I'll show you out."

Jacques Siethbüller got up and escorted them to his secretary's desk.

"Genevieve, can you schedule the bloodwork for Mr. and Mrs. Terebus and make another appointment for them in ten to fifteen days? I'll see you soon, and don't give up hope," he concluded.

Then he went back into his office.

∼

IN THE WINTER OF 1989, this is what Noemie wrote in her diary:

. . .

JANUARY 12, 1989,

After having thought it over, we decided to make an appointment with this famous specialist in Paris. Sacha chose Professor Siethbüller from Dr. Lepic's list: one of his colleagues told him that he was internationally recognized! Hallelujah!

More blood samples...
Seeding of lymphocytes...
Artificial blocking of cell divisions... High-power microscope analysis... Chromosomal photo slicing...
Classification of genes by pairs (the karyotype, a word I'd only heard before in the Telethon!
And finally the verdict, on the chopping block...

∼

JANUARY 22, **1989,**

HERE WE ARE. *We know the cause now. The chromosomal analysis has rendered its verdict, much worse than a sentence in a court of law.*

My genetic heritage has an anomaly making it impossible for an embryo to grow! This case is extremely rare and irreversible because it stems from what makes up my body: this genetic map that's like the unique and unfalsifiable ID card everyone has.

Sacha and I won't be able to naturally have a child together!

And what's more, is that whatever we do now, this child

will never have my genetic baggage, and it'll never really be mine...

So in these conditions, are we going to pursue our desire to have a child if it's not really ours?

Are we going to give up?

Rather than the tenacity of medically assisted procreation, wouldn't it be better to adopt a baby who was born at the wrong time in the wrong place?

All of these questions are bouncing around in our heads and hearts that for months now have been so strained.

We wanted to take time to think it over.

In the meanwhile, I reread some of the notes I'd written in my notebook a long time ago and I can measure how far we've come from then.

At that time I'd written 'happiness in starting a family,' 'this marvelous adventure,' 'this magical interlude' 'of nine months, maybe a year,' 'an unforgettable year,' 'a human adventure fulfilling all women...'

Today, nearly three years late (three years!!), it's like I couldn't have written these words myself. Where did all that optimism go, those beautiful words and that hope?

I wanted my testimonial to be an ode to the happiness of giving birth.

It's become a repository of our heartache, our difficulties and our doubts. It's now depressing, and I'd wanted it to sparkle with the light of a new life.

I can't do this anymore. These will be my last words, the last page of this journal. The cover will close on these sad words before they drag us down to the abyss of pain.

BUT LEO never read these last pages of suffering and disillusions, as she had ripped them out after having written them.

~

AT THE END OF JANUARY, 1989, they went to see Professor Siethbüller once again. He had the results of the tests that his genetics laboratory had carried out.

Sacha and Noemie were holding hands below the desk, eager to find out the medical verdict.

"I've got the results," the Professor began. "I'm not going to beat around the bush here, I much prefer to be as direct and as clear as possible: they don't look good."

The couple looked at each other, then at the doctor. He continued.

"But that doesn't mean your case is hopeless. Now listen closely: you can still have a child, but not in the old-fashioned way. Mrs. Terebus, your genetic heritage has a small anomaly making it impossible for an embryo to grow. But this anomaly doesn't prohibit you from having the fetus grow inside you later on."

"I don't get it, Professor," said Noemie, sobbing.

"I'll try to be clearer and spell it out. You have a very good chance of having a child if you use medically assisted procreation. But not with your own genes. On the other hand, you've got no problems Mr. Terebus. So you could have an oocyte that has been donated and you'd even be at the top of the list because your specific case is so rare."

"A donated oocyte?" Noemie said, surprised. "That means using another woman's genes?"

"That's right, an anonymous donation. The ovule of Mrs. X, mixed with your husband's sperm. So with this association, you'll obtain a viable fecundation, and then it will be implanted into your uterus. The embryo, which has now become a fetus, will continue its growth inside you."

"But that's with someone else's genes!"

"That's right, Mrs. Terebus, but just think the fetus will be growing inside you, you'll be the only person involved!"

"I don't know, I...," stuttered Noemie.

"Honey," Sacha said, trying to console her. "It's an opportunity for us."

"I understand your concerns," Siethbüller said. "I'm faced with this type of case nearly every day and I'm aware that it's a difficult decision for couples to make. You'll have to talk it over between yourselves. There are several associations that address these themes. If you want to join one, Genevieve can give you their details, maybe talking with other couples who have had the same decisions to make could help you."

"I thought... I believed..." Noemie sobbed.

"That you could... heal me... I don't know... make me function like a real woman."

"I'm sorry, but this discipline is still too young to accomplish this, or heal or repair something like your case. For right now, we can discover the problems in the chromosome, but we can't fix them. Maybe in a few decades. Right now our team and the Evry Genoscope - a French lab I'm proud of - are working to decipher the human genome. You have to be patient. But for you, the only solution is an oocyte donation or adoption. Think about it at home and come back and see me when you've made a decision, I'll take your case on personally."

Noemie and Sacha went back to Besancon with questions that were not the same as when they came to Paris, though they were still essential and hard to answer. Sacha favored an ovule donation, but Noemie, who would of course be the one receiving it, was far from agreeing with him. Quite on the contrary, that was something that deterred her, to the point that she didn't even want a baby anymore.

Chapter 42

Besançon, February, 1989

NOEMIE PUT her coat and shoes on and grabbed her bag from the coat rack. This was a Saturday afternoon in February.

Sacha was busy in his office, putting the final touches on a client study that he had to give to his boss on Monday.

She opened the door and shouted out to him.

"I'm going honey, have a good afternoon!"

"Thanks sweetie, where are you off to?"

"What a scatterbrain! I told you at noon. I'm going to Aline's because we're preparing a project for the ninth graders together."

"That's right, I remember now. Sorry, this file for our Spanish customer is overwhelming me here. Have a good afternoon gals!"

"Bye," said Noemie, running out.

"Bye," replied Sacha, to no one.

And he started working again on the project that would probably take most of the weekend to finish. Sometimes his boss asked him to work on engineering for his key clients. After all, he was an executive, he did work a lot, but he had substantial advantages: he thought he came out on the winning side of time against money. Sacha was trying to build up assets before a child would come and fill the house with his noise. And then once he'd become a father, he'd turn things around: less money but more time to spend with his family.

Noemie had left a good half-hour ago when the phone rang. There were two phones in the house: one in the living room and the other one right next to him on his desk. He picked up.

"Hello."

"Ah! Hi Sacha, it's Aline."

"Hi Aline. How you doing?"

"Fine! As always. What about you? You're not outside with this nice weather? You picked up as soon as I called so I'd imagine you're working, right?"

"That's it, Columbo! What can I do for you, beautiful lady?"

"I just wanted to ask Noemie something. Is she there?"

"No, she left about a half hour ago."

"Ah! It can wait till Monday then, I'll see her at school. Thanks Sacha."

"Wait a sec. I thought she was at your place.

"At my house? Um no, not yet... Aline hesitated.

"Strange she's not there yet. She must have been waylaid by a nice shop!"

"That's probably right, she'll be here soon. Man, am I ever absent-minded! Well, good luck if you're working then.".

"Okay, thanks and have fun working on your educational project too."

"The project... Right. That damn project," sputtered Aline. "All work, no play! See ya!"

And she hung up.

Sacha was pensive, listening to the indifferent tonality of the phone he was still holding. First of all he agreed that Aline was really absent-minded, a fully charged electric battery doing several things at the same time, and sometimes mixing them up. But for her to forget that her best friend was coming to work on a school project... That was strange. He hung up the phone. Then he surprised himself by thinking that maybe his wife had lied to him. When he thought back, he'd found her happier than usual to go out, as if she was trying to hide something else, a vexation perhaps. Recently Noemie had frequently been swinging from melancholy to euphoria, without any apparent reason for this. Her moods changed. Sometimes she seemed to be distant, lost in her secret thoughts.

He'd noticed that she went out more and more often on Saturday afternoons. And now, this supposed visit to Aline's, and this strange phone call.

Sacha had a mental image that disturbed him and he tried to get it out of his mind. Noemie had a lover and she'd gone to join him, that's why she'd been so strange lately.

This thought brought him back to Maeva. How could he blame his wife?

This baby that didn't come and this question of an oocyte donation which was now a taboo subject between them, starting to make them both go crazy... and maybe even do something foolish which could, in the long run, compromise their life as a couple.

Sacha went back to work, still musing. What would he do when she came back, start yelling at her? But if he did, he'd also have to admit his *mea culpa*.

Maybe the best idea was to keep it to himself. And to hope that a baby would soon come to sort out this sentimental mess.

Chapter 43

Sochaux, February, 2015

PIPPO SHOOK hands with the guy who had unloaded his semi.

"See you next time, little Italy," he said.

"*Ciao, Francese. Arrivederci*," Pippo answered as usual.

"Yeah, *arriva dirt she*," the little mustached guy joked, handing him his signed and sealed delivery slip.

This was a little ritual they shared.

Pippo climbed into his cab awkwardly. His knee was throbbing. He winced when he sat down on the comfortable seat. He slammed the door, blew onto his rugged hands, started up and slowly drove to the southern door of the PSA Peugeot-Citroën site in Sochaux.

The first time he'd come there he was amazed at how big this site was. The facility was a city in a city. To go from one entrance to another, you had to take a freeway! That time he had to go five extra miles to find the right entrance. Now he was used to this. An old-timer.

On the A36, he headed towards Besancon-Lyon. He'd planned on taking a little personnel detour and he had a mission to accomplish here. It was too late to turn back. She had to pay for it.

Pay for it, as she caused all his misfortunes, she was the cause of his failed life. She was the cause of those ten dark years he'd spent behind bars.

Everything started that night when she broke his knee. After that, things continued, each time plunging him even deeper into the darkest abyss.

His career was over. And his dreams too. He'd become violent, she fled.

He drank more and more to forget, but his knee, which had required long months of physical therapy, kept on reminding him of what had happened.

He flitted from one girl to another, perhaps an outlet to Her absence. But these new girls, from all walks of life and all over the world were mere pale copies. He sometimes even had to pay, to ease his body and conscience.

Alcohol, despair and bitterness soon led to an explosive cocktail, and Pippo became more and more violent as time went by.

He went from periods of withdrawal to deeper and deeper and more serious relapses.

When he was clean, he still seduced new women, but he too quickly started using again and just as quickly they ran off, terrorized by his uncontrollable rage.

Pippo started to be hauled off to police stations after several of them had filed complaints against him. More and more often he woke up in the grey dawn of drunk tanks.

Then one evening, when he'd had more alcohol than usual, plus had consumed certain drugs, he hit one of those women harder than usual or perhaps longer than usual, or in the wrong place.

That lady never got up again. He was sentenced to twelve years.

Judges had admitted attenuating circumstances, as he had been high on drugs.

Good conduct shaved two years off the sentence. Seemingly good conduct. Because behind Pippo's calm and sober mask, hatred was simmering.

Despite bullying by the other prisoners, he'd never fought back, he'd always accepted the unacceptable.

He didn't scream when the leader of the pack in Block 3 kept kicking him in his knee that was already fragile.

Hands clenching his steering wheel, Pippo

relived that scene, just as vividly as it was back in the Milan jail.

"You're gonna suffer now," sniggered the Block 3 leader, naked in the shared showers where Pippo found himself surrounded by a group of losers behind him. "You're ugly, Pippo! Take this!"

Pippo was lying on the tiles in the showers, water running in front of his eyes, making it hard to see. His assailants seemed like dark shadows, uncontrollable demons whose hatred targeted their poor consenting victim. He knew by experience that fighting back would be even worse, and that it was better to let them hit him and wait till the storm blew over. They'd get tired before him. A ragdoll wasn't as fun as an adversary who fought back.

The prison guards allowed this: they felt that the security and tranquility of the jailhouse was inversely proportional to the violence between prisoners! The more they settled their scores between themselves, the less problems they caused. They only butted in as a last resort, when they feared someone would die.

No one died today though.

Pippo had clenched his teeth for a few minutes, then the hyenas ran off, exhausted by his passivity.

The prison guards got him back up again, panting, dripping. Then they put a towel around him and took him to the infirmary.

He had a few hours, a few days of relative comfort, taken care of by the nurses whose gentleness contrasted with the ambient violence. He also spent a few weeks under strict surveillance at the Milan University Hospital after that.

He felt like he was traveling... like he was on vacation! Almost like he'd escaped.

Not just physically, but also mentally.

Ten years of thinking about the causes and *The* cause for his fall. Ten years of convincing himself that that *bitch*, the one who'd wrecked his life, had to pay the price.

Ten years of imagining what he'd do to avenge himself when he got out. How could he make her suffer too, just like she deserved... Pippo turned on his blinker and drove his thirty-eight-ton semi onto the Besancon-Palente exit. His day was nearly over, lamps were already lighting up the city. He was going to rest a while and then scout out the neighborhood.

Chapter 44

Milan, October, 2015

"AFTER THAT NIGHT when I told your father all about why I refused to have a child, months passed without us mentioning the subject again, though I knew that he'd never stopped thinking about starting a family. He'd understood my pain and he was resigned. In the meanwhile, with your mother, they still kept trying to have you. Whereas my psychological pain was lessening, his was little by little emerging, a bit stronger each time we saw each other in Milan. I could see him losing hope, he no longer had that sparkle in his eyes that characterized him and made him so loveable. So one day, after we'd made love tenderly, so he wouldn't irremediably sink into despair, I decided to do something about it."

∽

MILAN, **March, 1989**

"*AMORE MIO*, I'll give you that child you want so much!"

"Come on Maeva, you know it's impossible. I can't have a child with you, my mistress, and keep on living that sterile hell with my wife. How could I ever look at myself in the mirror each morning, without cursing my selfishness?"

"That wasn't what I meant, dear. Either you didn't understand me or I wasn't clear enough. I already told you: I don't want to be a mother, all that is *finito* for me. No, what I'm proposing here is to give your wife what she doesn't have and what I don't need anymore!"

"You're scaring me here... You mean... You'd be a porter for my wife's genes and my own?"

"Ah no! Can you imagine me, completely deformed, eight months pregnant? A huge stomach, greasy skin, stretch marks on my stomach, cellulite on my hips and butt, throwing up, and I'm sure I forgot the best! And then have a child, give it to your wife and I'd be the one with stretch marks, hanging tits and a huge butt? No, *grazie*!"

"So what's your idea then?"

"It's easy. You told me that your wife's problem was that her ovaries couldn't expulse any oocytes? So the problem is located right at the beginning of the chain. If your wife found that missing link, after that there wouldn't be any problems?"

"That's what the specialists say, at least that Siethbüller guy you advised me to see."

"Oh! You finally went then? You convinced your wife?"

"Yes. We saw him in January."

"So? What did you think of him?"

"Very professional, very gentle, easy to talk to."

"But he still didn't convince your wife, that's the problem?"

"She still doesn't want to hear anything about a donated oocyte. She refuses to have the genes of an unknown person inside her, or should I say that the baby would have genes that weren't hers."

"And if these genes that weren't hers were mine?" Sacha gaped at her for a long while, lost in his thoughts.

"You're scaring me again. How can you give us your genes? Wrap them up and tie a ribbon around them?"

"Don't be such an idiot, Sacha. I'm serious. I'd like to be the one giving you this beautiful gift. Because, in my own way, I love you. And also, and it's strange I know, but I also appreciate your wife, I sympathize with your disillusions, and I only want the best for both of you. I'm giving you myself, I'm giving you a life... What do you think?"

"I love this idea but it's completely crazy. An oocyte donation is anonymous, meaning that your idea is totally unrealistic and undoable! Even if you donated your oocyte in the facility where my wife would be implanted with a fertilized egg, you'd have like one chance out of…I have no idea… that the interventions would match! With all the manipulations there must be. But it is very generous of you."

"I know all that Sacha. If you trust me, I think I can get around all these hurdles."

"Really? How? Would you break in at night like a medically assisted procreation Arsene Lupin to find your sample and mix it with mine?"

"Be serious for two minutes, *Caro Mio*. I'm thinking of Professor Siethbüller. You could say that he's a bit more than just a simple professional acquaintance."

"A friend?"

"A bit more, a bit less, according..."

"You mean you've been intimate with him?"

"We were... we still are a little, every once in a while."

"You're sleeping with him? asked Sacha, offended. "You are really a..."

"Listen up," Maeva interrupted him. "You're not the best example of a faithful husband. So please just shut up and listen to me! Professor Siethbüller owes me, or anyway does whatever I ask him to: he's crazy about me. I have to fly to Paris in a couple of days, I'll go and see him."

"I understand. But the hardest part is yet to come: convincing him to ignore his Hippocratic oath by doing what you've planned out in your little head."

"That's no problem for me. Jacques is a married man too and I don't think that he'd appreciate his wife finding out that he's got a soft spot for young beautiful Italians... Just tell me if you're convinced by my idea that your child would have my genes, and I'll take care of things behind the scene."

Sacha thought about her proposal. He finally answered.

"It's crazy from a deontological and human point of view, but I think I like it."

"So one more thing, handsome: now you've got to convince your wife to accept the donation or in other words, carry my genes."

Chapter 45

Paris, March, 1989

MAEVA WENT into the elevator of the Concorde Lafayette Hotel, right next to the Porte-Maillot *Palais des Congrès*, a masterpiece of modern architecture, only about ten years old, and just as high as the famous Tour Montparnasse.

The ride up was quick and comfortable. A few men wearing suits and ties and a couple of young smartly dressed women were with her.

The young Italian went up to the thirty-fourth floor where the Panoramic Bar overlooking the capital was located.

She walked in, admiring the fantastic view of Paris from each window. She looked around to find the man she was meeting here.

He came up to her with a smile on his face.

White teeth, salt and peppered hair carefully parted on the side.

"Maeva, you're even more beautiful than the view of the City of Light!"

"*Buongiorno Professore*! What a beautiful place, you're right, I've never been here."

"Did you know we're nearly four hundred feet high? What would you like to drink?"

"A Martini, of course, even if we're not in Milan."

"Barman. A *Martini Bianco* for the beautiful lady and a glass of your best champagne for me. We'll be sitting over here," Professor Siethbüller said to the employee.

He put a hand on Maeva's back to delicately show her to the two comfortable armchairs next to the picture window overlooking the Eiffel Tower.

"How's your conference?" said Maeva sitting down.

"Really good. So as you can see, this venue is perfect, with a direct access to the *Palais* from the hotel. The laboratories are really generous with me, they booked me a magnificent suite on the twenty-sixth floor with a view of the *Bois de Boulogne* and Roland Garros tennis courts. Plus, icing on the cake, here you are with me. I must admit I was surprised you called."

"Yes, I wanted to see you. I'm leaving on Sunday from Orly, I've got a room at the Sofitel Arch of Triumph."

"Plenty of room in my suite you know," the professor whispered to her while the barman served their drinks. "Put it on my tab, please."

"Of course, sir. If you'll just sign here."

Maeva took a sip of her Martini on the rocks.

"Your wife isn't joining you this time?" she asked casually while looking out over the Parisian rooftops.

"You know Annie is really busy with all her associations, her volunteer work, plus her university courses. She decided to go back to school and she's studying for a bachelor's degree in psychology! At her age..." he said ironically while looking at Maeva's cleavage.

"Maybe she's bored? You know, a professor's wife: your work at the hospital, your courses at the university, your seminars all over the world, including Milan for the past five years. Maybe you're not there enough for her so she compensates by filling up her agenda."

"She's got everything she could ever want: a beautiful house in Paris, another one in Biarritz, an apartment in Megève, another one on the Costa Del Sol, Chanel clothing, her own car, you name it."

Maeva nodded, smiling.

"My poor Jacques, even though you're an intelligent and brilliant professor, you don't understand a thing about human psychology, and feminine psychology even less so. You're the one who should be taking courses at the university!"

"Don't be cheeky, Maeva, leave my wife out of this. So why this surprise visit?"

Maeva took another sip of her martini.

"I'd like you to do something for me."

Jacques Siethbüller squinted at her over his nearly empty glass of champagne.

"I'm listening. It's not a problem with your health I hope. "You look wonderful."

"No, no, don't worry, I'm fine. Actually it's sort of a delicate situation, it's not for me and yes, it is linked to health. Or at least related to the medical field, that's why I thought maybe you could help me here."

"You need a consultation from a specialist? You'd like to take advantage of the knowledge the Great Professor in Medicine has," he continued.

"Stop it, you arrogant French rooster!" Maeva said with a smile. "Let's be serious. It's complicated enough as it is. It's for a friend, someone French, like you."

"Hmmm. You're specializing in French guys now?"

"Quit being ironic and just listen to me. This man has a problem with his wife."

"So he's married too?"

"Right, and he loves his wife. They want to have a child, they've been trying for ages, but nothing works. They've already had loads of exams, but there doesn't seem to be a solution for them. So I had an idea, as you're a specialist in this recent technique, what's its name already? MAP?"

"That's it, medically assisted procreation. That's what this seminar is about. So what's their problem? Is it his fault? Or hers? Or both of them?

"Apparently it's hers. Some problem with her tubes or ovaries, I don't really know."

"Where do they live?

"In Besancon, I think. But they already took all the tests over there and the doctors said they can't do anything for them: they have to consult a top specialist."

"Like the one in Paris, the famous Professor Siethbüller?"

"That would be a solution."

Jacques Siethbüller looked at the Arch of Triumph in the background. He seemed to be thinking it over.

"It's true that we're benchmarks in genetic research as well as one of Europe's best sites for difficult medically assisted procreation cases. What would you like me to do? Get them a quick appointment with me?"

"They're so unhappy. They're dreaming of having a baby, one that has been conceived naturally... or should I say they don't really agree about this. To tell you the truth, my friend is ready to benefit from a donation of egg cells for his wife, so he can see her little stomach grow and grow and finally have a baby, but she's reluctant to accept someone else's genes."

Maeva sighed.

"It makes me sad for them."

Jacques caressed her hand that was on the round table next to her glass of martini.

"It looks like their problem really affects you."

"It does. Sacha - that's the name of my friend - is someone really dear to me and I feel like I understand his wife, by proxy."

"By proxy? You mean you don't know her?"

"That's right. I've never met her, but after all these years, I feel like I know her."

"Okay. Maeva, I don't want to pry, but I've got the impression you're hiding something from me. This Sacha guy, he's just a friend or…?"

Maeva bit her bottom lip.

"A bit more than a friend."

"A friend like me?"

"No, Jacques, not a friend like you."

"Meaning?"

"Yes, I'm his mistress. His too. You know I'm not exclusive. But it was really different with him. First it was love at first sight, then the feeling that I understood him, I shared his heartaches and his joys, his desires. And I really want to help him, viscerally."

"You are wonderful when you're in love *Cara*. You take men, you help yourself, you're like a praying mantis. At the same time though, you're a

Saint-Bernard, a first-aider, a Good Samaritan for feelings. Another glass?"

"Yes, thanks."

"Waiter! The same thing, please."

They didn't speak while the waiter took their glasses and served them a second round. Jacques then continued the discussion.

"It seems to me that it's not really a medical issue here, it's a problem between both of them. If they don't agree, I can't do anything for them. We can't force them, it's delicate. What am I supposed to do here? What do you really want from me?"

Maeva got up from her armchair, as if she was embarrassed by how this conversation was going. She wanted to say more but was uncomfortable doing so. She finally answered.

"It's a bit more complicated than that. I've got an idea... maybe it's crazy, but I'd like to run it through you. I'm counting on your sense of altruism and understanding."

"Wow. I'm starting to get worried here by words like that. Let me finish my champagne."

Acting on his words, Jacques finished his bubbly and sat back in his armchair, ready to hear what Maeva had to tell him.

"Here we go then," she said, looking Siethbüller right in the eyes, "my request will seem absurd to you, but it's something that makes sense to me and will benefit everyone: Sacha, his wife Noemie, and equally myself, as a woman."

Professor Siethbüller was disturbed when he heard those first names which, attached to the city of Besancon she'd mentioned earlier, seemed to ring a bell. Though he had a skeptical frown, he didn't interrupt Maeva.

"You know, Jacques, we already talked about when I lost my baby a couple of years ago with that soccer star. Anyway, Sacha is already convinced. If that's the way it would happen, he agrees."

"What did you guys already agree to?" asked Jacques Siethbüller, massaging his temples with the migraine that suddenly had hit him. "Here you're not worrying me anymore, you're scaring me!"

"Listen, Jacques, try to understand. I know, it's crazy, it's even incredible you could say, but it's a conviction. I always wanted a child, but that didn't work out for me. Plus, I do love Sacha. Almost like a brother, actually. And I want to give him what he wants the most: a child, this child, their child."

"Well, just do it then! He wouldn't be the first man to divorce his sterile wife for his fertile mistress," he said dryly.

"Sacha would never leave his wife! Plus I would never ask him to. I'm not designed to have a husband, a child, a family. I need my freedom, to sleep with who I want to, when I want to, like with you, for example."

"Trying to butter me up here," said the professor ironically. "Speaking of which, we haven't seen each other often lately."

Maeva caressed his cheek delicately.

"Maybe we can work something out... If you help me!"

"Blackmail! But tempting. Maeva, when I see you, I want you so much. My suite is just downstairs. How about continuing this little discussion there?"

"No, you wouldn't concentrate. Let me finish my line of thought. What I mean is this child, I'd like to have it with Sacha, with Noemie. I'd like to donate my genes, my oocytes."

"You are completely crazy, that's all I can say! You know that any donation of egg cells is completely anonymous and free. And when you say free, it means that there are no personal interests or calculations. Do you actually realize what you're asking of me?"

"I know Jacques, I'm asking what's unimaginable, crazy, impossible."

"That's it: impossible. Without even mentioning medical ethics!

"I know all that. That's all I've been thinking about, night after night. I know we're talking about human lives here. And that's important."

"Listen, just relax. Anyway, your plan isn't going to work and there's nothing for me to do in it. Technically speaking, I have my hands tied, I can't even influence anyone even as head of their department. I'm a professor in medicine, not a lab technician dammit!"

"Jacques, please don't get mad. It's already so hard.

"I'm not mad, I just think you're insane and that your dumb idea is not going to work. Forget it."

Maeva turned her face towards the windows and silently looked out at the large Parisian boulevards below the Lafayette Tower. She looked at the cars, listened to the murmurs of the city, attenuated by the altitude and double-glazed windows. A tear dropped from her left eye and she spoke to Jacques, without looking at him, or perhaps it was just to herself.

"I want to do something good. I want to make three people happy by just a simple donation of an infinitely small part of myself."

Jacques got up and caressed her nape while she kept on looking outside.

"I have to go back to the Conference; I'll be speaking in half an hour. Here's the key to my suite, twenty-fourth floor, room 2451. Why don't you rest there and I'll join you later, okay?"

"No, Jacques, I prefer to wander around in Paris, go to the shops, maybe a museum, sit down in a park, rather than brooding on this."

"Well, in that case, how about coming with me to the gala cocktail tonight that Bayer is organizing? Eight o'clock on the first floor of the *Palais*."

"Alright, but please think about what I asked you."

Jacques Siethbüller sighed.

"I think I've already made up my mind."

They left the panoramic bar together and walked to the elevators. They were alone inside, Jacques took Maeva's hand and turned towards her for a quick kiss. She turned her head.

"Not now, Jacques. Maybe later."

"You blame me for not being able to help you?"

The elevator doors opened and they went out. In the lobby Maeva rummaged around in her bag and took out a photo she handed to Jacques.

"Take a look, these are the people I'm talking about. Look at their eyes." Professor Siethbüller stammered.

"I know them."

"They're the ones I sent to you and you had an appointment with them in January."

"You can tell they're in love. But feelings and genetics don't work well together. See you tonight then?"

"*Ciao*!" said Maeva, walking across the huge lobby towards the exit.

The sun was shining that afternoon in Paris, but Maeva's heart was overcast, full of doubts and painful twinges. That afternoon the Palais des Congrès was noisy and joyful, but Jacques was elsewhere, full of questions and absurd thoughts.

Chapter 46

Paris, March 1989, End of the day

THEY GOT BACK TOGETHER in the evening in the main amphitheater where Professor Siethbüller was finishing up his presentation on the most recent developments in genetics in the field of gynecology.

"My dear colleagues, I thank you for your attention during this long presentation. As you saw, now our specialization is significant, thanks to the sequencing of the human genome and the Evry Genoscope is a benchmark in the industry. I'd also like to sincerely thank its president, Mr. Jean-Philippe Talbot, who, thanks to his pugnacity, his dynamics and also thanks to the financial support of the Ministry of Research and many generous donors through this marvelous operation called the

Telethon, will allow even more new and key discoveries."

The president got up from his seat in the front row and turned to face the pool of doctors in the amphitheater, who warmly applauded him.

"Thank you," said Siethbüller, covering the nourished applause. "And now we'd like to invite you for the gala cocktail dinner sponsored by Takeda Laboratory on the third floor. Make sure you have your badge. Thank you all very much and see you again next year at the same place, about the same date, and I hope with more new scientific discoveries for our specializations."

The audience applauded him. In the back of the room, Maeva admired the professor. He'd obtained a guest badge for her so she'd be able to join him for cocktails. He liked to be seen with charming "colleagues" hanging on to his arm. After having shook hands with several doctors, and while the amphitheater was slowly emptying, he walked up to her.

"I'm so happy you decided to come," he whispered.

"I've got a role to play," she replied ironically. "Did you have time to think about what we talked about?"

Siethbüller sighed.

"I was going to, but I didn't have time to. But I will, I promise."

"The earlier the better, you know that the biological clock keeps on ticking…"

They went up to the third floor together, had a few appetizers and a couple of glasses of champagne while working the floor, chatting with guests and scientists, conversations that were interesting for him but boring for her. She nonetheless kept on smiling, playing her role as Great Professor Siethbüller's companion, the great master of gynecological genetics, respected by his peers.

Professor Edwige Mazarico joined them.

"Jacques, your wife isn't here this year?"

A question asked while glancing at Maeva who perfectly understood the innuendo. Something women could do easily.

"No, she had so much to do with all her associations, you know."

Professor Mazarico was a short stout little lady with twinkling eyes.

"I understand, doing volunteer work is so rewarding. I admire people like her who spend their time helping others. Can you introduce us?" she asked, looking at Maeva.

"Of course," Siethbüller answered. "This is Maeva D'Annunzio, an Italian friend who's passing through Paris. Maeva, this is Professor Edwige Mazarico, she specializes in embryology."

Both ladies smiled.

"Are you a doctor too?" Mazarico asked.

"Not at all," replied Maeva laughing.

"Maeva's a flight attendant for Alitalia. And I actually met her a couple of years ago when I was flying to Rome."

"It must be exciting traveling all the time, all around the world."

"When you first start, it is. But quite quickly, like in any job I'd imagine, it becomes a routine and starts to get boring. Plus we don't always have enough time to visit all the beautiful monuments. Sometimes stopovers are really short and we just want to go home. Without forgetting all the jetlag, brutal changes in weather conditions, different food, and all that. Plus we always have to keep on smiling!"

"And I must say that you do have a nice smile. I understand that Jacques appreciates your company when you're in Paris, Miss or Mrs...?"

"Miss," Maeva answered.

"Nice to have met you," said the professor with a new wry smile. "Have a good stay here. I have to go because I see Takeda's CEO over there and I have to talk to him before he leaves. I'll call you soon, Jacques. I'd like to tell you about a study I read about in The Lancet, I'm sure you'd be interested in it."

"We'll talk on Monday then. See you soon, Edwige."

She quickly walked away. Maeva took advantage of this to whisper into the professor's ear.

"Looks like someone has a reputation here. This

Edwige seems to insinuate that you're usually in good company. I would suppose that your wife doesn't suspect a thing or else she just ignores it."

"My wife, you know all she wants from me is that I bring in the money so she can live the life she wants without working," Siethbüller said ironically.

"My dear Jacques, you don't understand a thing about women. I wonder what she'd think about our affair?"

"Why did you say that?"

"Oh. Just like that. But if you don't decide to help me out with what we talked about earlier...

"What? After blackmail, now you're threatening me?"

"Not really. Just a little friendly advice. Sometimes women talk too much, put their feet in their mouths…"

While speaking, they left the amphitheater, went down to the lobby and walked towards the Concorde Lafayette Hotel through the luxury shopping gallery.

"Maeva, what you're asking me is dicey. It's illegal and doesn't comply with our rules of professional conduct."

"Jacques, they need your help!" replied Maeva. "We both can make them happy."

"Let's continue this conversation in my suite. It'll be more comfortable," insisted Siethbüller, hugging her.

"I bet you've got something else in mind," she said, laughing.

"Not just in mind," added Jacques, sliding his hand down her back and onto her buttocks.

She pulled it away.

"No, don't touch. You have to deserve it."

"By doing what?"

"Maybe by being really nice to me," whispered Maeva. "Indulging me… and then maybe I can indulge you too."

"Hmm. Are you talking about this story of oocytes again? Jesus Maeva, it's crazy and you know it. Don't count on it. First of all, your friends don't need me to have a donation of egg cells: they've got the right to it and the donation is anonymous, so there isn't anything preventing them from doing it."

They reached the elevator they'd taken earlier in the day from the panoramic bar on the 34th floor. This time Siethbüller pushed button 24.

"I know all that," continued Maeva, taking Jacques' hand. "But if they're not my genes, they won't do it. You already met them, you know she's not really in favor of this method. This equation is simple: they're unhappy, to make them happy they need a child, and this child can only be obtained through an artificial method. Me, I've got oocytes that no one's using, and I want to donate them. I convinced Sacha and he'll convince Noemie."

"So if I understand what you're getting at: they'll use your genes and they'll do the IVF because Sacha will secretly be privy to what's going on, or they won't do a thing and they'll never have a child?"

The elevator door opened and they walked to room 2451. Siethbüller opened it, they walked into the suite and he locked the door.

"That's right, Jacques. I know it's crazy, but all four of us are required for them to be happy: Noemie, Sacha, you, and myself, at different levels. Some people will know stuff the others won't but at the end of the day, it will be a good deed, a very good deed!"

"Good, but rigged, and not exactly kosher."

While he was speaking Jacques was playing with Maeva's dress. Her sparkling dress had a zipper in the front to adjust how high or low her cleavage should be. Before going to the Convention, the young lady had zipped it barely above her breasts. Siethbüller was playing with the zipper and her breasts were right below the opening.

"It's just a little gesture for you to do for a marvelous result for this couple," Maeva insisted.

Siethbüller's breathing accelerated as the zipper descended. His eyes were sparkling with excitement, in anticipation.

"A tiny manipulation," she continued. "Fate's little helping hand."

The professor kneeled down in front of Maeva. The zipper was open to her navel. Swathes of her dress were falling with each new inch: you could already see her breasts, only her nipples were holding the fabric up. Jacques was panting.

"There's no risk for you, no one will see you, and it will only take a minute," Maeva insisted, running her fingers through the doctor's hair while he was kissing the sensitive zone of skin between the top of her panties and her navel.

"Please Jacques, do it for me."

Siethbüller grumbled a few intelligible words while continuing to kiss her skin. Then he raised his arms, took hold of the two straps and slid them down over her shoulders. Her small and proud breasts emerged entirely and the professor's powerful hands seized them.

She suddenly moved back three steps. The dress fell down and all she was wearing now were her black panties.

"Jacques, answer me. Are you going to help me?"

"Come back!" he belched out, still kneeling, excited beyond control. "I want you."

"If you give me your word. If you help me I'll do whatever you want, as often as you want."

"Ah! Little devil! You're driving me crazy!"

He got up and neared her, his mouth and hands wanting more. She backed up to the edge of the king-sized bed.

"You'll do it?"

"Maybe," he whispered, taking her in his arms. "If you do what you know I love, you know…"

"Yes, I know. I know your little delicious weakness," said Maeva, getting out of his arms and walking around him. She forced him to sit down on the bed and then she kneeled down in front of his legs spread open. She expertly undid his belt and then the buttons on his Armani suit. The professor was already quite excited by the thought of what was to come. His trousers slid down his legs and calves to his polished shoes.

"I won't take '*Maybe*' as an answer," Maeva warned him, running her nails over his thighs.

"Keep on, keep on."

Maeva took his erect sex and began to delicately masturbate him.

"Ah! Little devil," he repeated without much imagination. "You know how to butter up a man!"

"Tell me that you'll do what I asked you, Jacques." She approached her lips. Her long hair hid her face, but Jacques guessed and knew what she was about to do.

"Okay, but don't stop and just shut up!"

She couldn't have spoken anyway, it would have been impolite.

A few instants later, Siethbüller, still sitting on the edge of the bed, shouted out amidst a series of spasms.

"Yes... yes... oh yes... okay... yes..." before falling back onto the bed.

Chapter 47

Paris, May, 1989

SACHA WAS SITTING on a plastic seat with the other men and women in the samples, donations and inseminations waiting room.

He was holding an old *Paris Match* magazine, mechanically turning the pages, barely looking at the photos. He thought of their slogan: *The weight of words, the shock of photos.*

He said to himself that his words finally had enough weight to convince Noemie.

Of course, he couldn't tell her why he himself had finally decided to accept a donation of egg cells, but he was able to tilt the playing field in the right direction. He'd found the decisive arguments so that Noemie accepted it. She hadn't bought into it immediately, but she finally admitted that the most important thing wasn't the genes of so and so, but the nine months she'd have being pregnant, these forty-three so very important weeks during which her baby would grow, nourish itself and flourish day after day in a total osmosis with its mother's body. The anonymous ovule would just be a helping hand, a spark that would light a joyful fire within her. Noemie was once again smiling and progressing.

That's how they both came for an appointment that would follow Sacha's sperm collection.

Sacha put down the faded *Paris Match*, glanced at his watch, picked up an old copy of *Auto-Plus* and then looked towards the restrooms to see if Noemie was coming out.

Noemie flushed the toilet, left and went towards the sinks to wash her hands and comb her hair. At the same time another woman walked out of one of the toilets and went to the neighboring sink for the same thing.

They both politely greeted each other and Noemie thought she'd heard a slight accent without being able to identify its origin. As their faces were both reflected in the large mirror above the sinks, Noemie had to admit that she was a very beautiful woman: long brown hair, slightly almond-shaped eyes and delicate and pulpy lips. She sort of looked like herself, except that she was a bit taller. Nicer looking though, she thought, with a twinge of jealousy. She even said to herself that had she been a man, she would have been attracted to the brunette.

Then she looked away from her and finished putting on her lipstick. The other lady was putting her hair up.

Noemie refreshed her lipstick as if the color in her heart and head had also been refreshed since she'd finally given into the idea of using a donation of egg cells from someone she didn't know. She was going to be a mother and tough luck if she wasn't at the origin of the process. What was most important was to raise the baby, educate it, support it, for the nine months *in utero* and then when he was a kid, a teen, and even into adulthood sometimes. It was the nature or nurture question, procreation and education. What was the most important thing in life: the second where the gametes met, or an entire life of love given by parents who loved each other and who showed this?

She put her lipstick back into her purse, smiled at the other lady, who smiled back at her. Noemie found her strangely malicious. She finally dared to speak up.

"Do we know each other? I think I've seen you somewhere."

The unknown lady seemed troubled by this question.

"I don't think so," replied Maeva. "I'm Italian and I don't come to France very often."

Noemie became emboldened by this girl-to-girl talk.

"You're here for medically assisted procreation too?"

"Sort of," she replied, lying. "I came with a friend who is going to receive a donation. You know it's not easy, so I came to support her."

"You're not kidding! My husband and I have been trying for years to find a solution and we finally decided to use this method too. With all the consequences that it implies."

"I'm sure things will go well for you. Plus, once you'll be holding your little baby, all your doubts, your fears and everything that you had to endure will disappear in a snap of your fingers! All these years will just be like a bad dream that has blown away."

Noemie felt relieved by these words and her soft, lilting voice.

"You're right, you have to have a positive attitude to increase your chances of succeeding."

"Exactly! Happiness is a choice too. Whatever you're up against, everyone is free to choose to be happy or to be unhappy."

"Thank you, your optimism was just what I needed! Funny place to meet, isn't it?"

"Right, well, good luck!"

"Thanks. And good luck to your friend too."

Noemie adjusted her purse on her shoulder,

went out of the restrooms and joined Sacha in the waiting room.

Maeva had immediately recognized the woman who was washing her hands. She'd seen a photo of her. Noemie, her lover's wife. They'd politely greeted each other and while arranging her hair, she'd noticed how she was looking at her, curiously and strangely with a touch of jealousy. Women were so clairvoyant. Had she only known who she was! And the role she'd played in all of this.

Maeva was happy for both of them. She'd be giving them a priceless gift, one they couldn't give themselves. She finally was going to do something. Her brief passage on Earth would not have been for nothing. Her adventure with Sacha would now have a true meaning, not just two people who had slept together for a couple of months. It was totally unexpected, but somehow, Sacha had gotten closer to Noemie when he'd met Maeva.

To some degree she'd saved their marriage and now was giving them hope to start a family.

She'd decided that after this, she could no longer be Sacha's mistress. She was going to tell him this and was sure that he'd also understand it and that he'd probably reached the same conclusion. They could still see each other, but as friends. With, despite everything, a permanent and living link between them... the child who would be born.

Noemie had suddenly spoken to her, politely, innocently. They'd exchanged a few sentences and

Sacha's wife only understood them in the first degree. Maeva had been nice to her. For a split second she'd thought about spilling the beans, but that would have spoiled everything! Instead of that she preferred to tell a little white lie. She'd conveyed her enthusiasm to her and felt *de facto*, happy about their future joy.

Maeva came out of the restrooms a bit after Noemie.

In the waiting room, she exchanged a brief wink with Sacha, who lovingly took his wife's hand. She could tell they were in love and she didn't want to spoil this.

Sacha had had a movement of dissimulated panic when he saw Maeva coming out of the restrooms. He suddenly realized she must have seen Noemie in there. They'd spent quite a bit of time in the restrooms. And if Maeva, whose smile suddenly seemed ironic to him when she came out, had told Noemie everything. No, that wasn't possible. You don't talk to unknown people in a hospital's restrooms to tell them about their husband's antics! Though Maeva was sometimes unpredictable, Sacha was sure that she'd never do a thing like that. Why would she have done it anyway? For revenge? She was the one who had instigated this assisted procreation deal, she wasn't going to spoil everything now! Everything was clear for all the parties present. Sacha tried to chase away those crazy ideas and to reassure himself and show his wife how much he loved her, he took her hand while his ex-mistress went to the back of the large room, disappearing behind one of the folding screens that separated the hall into several more intimate spaces.

He persuaded himself that he'd have to stop playing this stupid game, one that was unhealthy for everyone. Though he was in love with both women, he had to make a choice, and this choice was now clear to him: he wanted to become an involved, respectful and complete father. He knew that if he went back to Milan, their relationship would have changed: a strange form of friendship mixed with a strange genetic link would replace their former adulterous relation. Maeva had been a benediction, a gift of God, yes, a gift, that was the right word.

Professor Siethbüller crossed the waiting room to go to the medically assisted procreation room. He first looked at Maeva, then a few chairs away, in another section, at Sacha and Noemie, holding hands. He nodded at them and they smiled back.

Chapter 48

Milan, October, 2015

"YOU COULD SAY I'm the living proof that my dad finally succeeded in convincing my mom!"

"Yes, he did. It must have been so important to him that he knew what arguments he'd need."

"Still, if you look at Mom's notebooks, she'd completely abandoned this project of medical assistance."

"I know she didn't like the idea of carrying a child that wasn't genetically hers. Your father told me that she'd feel like she was carrying another person's child, like it was a foreign object inside her."

"Yes, but the embryo would have had Dad's genes! Already a success."

"I guess that's what tipped the scales. And I even

think that maybe your dad threatened to leave her if she didn't try this solution. I'm sure he never would have done it, but it must have borne its fruits because here you are!"

"So you got the green light to approach this coveted complacent professor?"

"I did and I called Professor Siethbüller the next day!"

"I know that name!" Leo said excitedly waiting to hear the rest. "He's one of France's leading specialists in medically assisted procreation. But I'm a little afraid to understand what you're saying here: you ended up convincing him to fiddle with my parents' medically assisted procreation process?"

"Well, for me everything was clear: you father was madly in love with your mother, your mother loved your father and both of them wanted a child, at any price. And I was the one who paid the price."

"You mean you bribed Professor Siethbüller? That's despicable!" the young man said.

"No, don't worry, no money changed hands. Just comprehension from that doctor who did disavow his medical ethics and principles because of the love and despair he'd seen in your parents' eyes. And I didn't hesitate for a single second. All the ingredients were there to make our idea work: your parents who were so in love, the strong relationship I had with your father, Professor Siethbüller's compassion, your mom's sterility and my unused fertility. So all that had to be done was mix all these ingredients up in the bottom of a test tube so everyone could be happy!"

Leo drank in all these secrets looking down into the bottom of his glass of champagne, wondering where all those bubbles came from, those light and sparkling ones that rose to the top. He smiled when he thought about the similarity between the test tube and glass of champagne.

"So I'm a test-tube baby then!"

"Exactly! But that doesn't exclude all the love we all had."

"You had to go to France for the oocyte extraction?"

"Yes, I did have to go back to your city. Not long at all, just a couple of hours in the hospital where I ran across your mother."

"You two met each other?"

"You could say that. To tell you the truth, we saw each other in the restroom while washing our hands. Or powdering our noses, like we say! We even said a few words to each other, small talk between two people. I'd recognized her as I'd already seen pictures of her. But she never knew who I was, that would have been uncomfortable, don't you think?"

"Uncomfortable for my dad you mean!"

"Probably. He knew I was there. I was completely serene though. Seeing them sitting next to each other, holding hands, almost looking each other in the eyes, I just knew I had made the right decision. I considered myself to be the cement holding them together rather than a destructive element as your father's 'mistress.' I was the missing link, the last piece of the puzzle they were doing."

"Like my dad said, there technically was one chance out of "X" possibilities that your oocyte would be fertilized by his genes and then injected into your mom. Except of course, unless the famous Professor Siethbüller in person took action."

"And that's exactly what happened! The professor made sure he was there the day they harvested my eggs and put a tiny but distinctive sign on the test tube so he could find it to mix it with your father's gametes. Before that though, you realize there are a whole series of manipulations to be done, including of course, the fusion between the male and female gametes. And that's what the professor did, simply and without ever having any of the lab technicians suspect a thing."

"I would imagine that as he was the head of the department he could do all these manipulations? You sure got the right person! It would have been more complicated with a simple technician, wouldn't it?"

"Of course. But as luck would have it, I knew this professor! Ah! this word 'luck.' The luck that followed you all through your life my little Leo, beginning with your conception."

"Pure chance. A lottery," Leo thought out loud.

"But a rigged lottery! So if I understand you, I'm nothing more than a mouse in a laboratory!"

"If that's what you think, you didn't understand a thing, nor what your mother wrote in her diary, nor what your father told you on the CD he'd left you, nor even what I just told you. You're much more than that, Leo! You're the fruit of love between three people when so many kids are born to a couple who doesn't love each other anymore, or to parents who don't love them and finally give them up. Your parents always loved you and even today, even if they're no longer here, they proved it to you by unveiling all these secrets and still are proving it, here and now, through myself!"

Maeva had raised her voice here, as if Leo's reaction revolted her. It was so important to her that Leo would admit his father's decision, as irrational as it was. Tears welled up in her eyes.

"Leo, I'd like you to know that I'm ready to return the love that your parents had for you and that until the day I die."

Leo looked at this lady's clouded eyes, someone he didn't know just a few days before, but who said that she was ready to play a part either in his heart, or at least in his personal story. This sixty-year-old lady who was so beautiful. This lady who - and now he was convinced of it - had the same nose he did, this little detail that had jumped out at him this morning when he was shaving, and that confirmed so visibly what she had told him. This lady who, far from replacing the mother he'd lost and who had raised him, was the person whose genes he shared and who said she'd play the role that she had never - in her whole life - wanted to play, that of his mother. Maeva looked at him.

"Now, I'm here for you, if you want this. Maybe I'm not your mother, but you'll always be a part of me."

Chapter 49

Geneva, Cointrin Airport, October, 2015

LEO SAW Aline who was waiting for him in the arrival's hall, behind the windows. He waved at her and she smiled back. His mother's best friend had agreed to pick him up at the airport as Chloe had already started her classes and on Wednesday, she was at the university.

"Hey Aline," said Leo, kissing her on the cheek in the way people did in their region: a frank kiss on one cheek and the other person did the same thing. Just one kiss each, but a real one, not some air-kiss!

"Did you have a good trip?"

"Fine, with Alitalia. Their flight attendants are top! Thanks for coming to pick me up."

"No problem. You know I'm here for you, and

Serge too of course, if you need anything. Whenever possible, of course. Would you like to come for supper one of these days with Chloe? I'll make something simple, it'll be casual, just so we can spend a little time together and you won't feel so alone."

"That's nice," Leo interrupted her, already smiling to see that Aline was still a chatterbox, almost hard to stop her once she'd started. "That'll be fun, I'll ask Chloe and we'll schedule a date. Where are you parked?"

"Third floor underground. Geneva Airport is really practical, it's almost like you park on the runway. It's not any farther from Besancon than Saint-Exupéry, but at least you're not parked miles away, you don't have to hop on a shuttle and if it's raining you don't get wet. Plus the parking lot is clean, safe, and functional with little green lamps that indicate free slots. It's Switzerland, what else can I say?"

While continuing to talk, Aline paid at the automatic pay station despite Leo's protests and pressed the button on the elevator. They went in and went down to the floor where her car was parked, an elegant and nervous Mini Cooper Countryman. Just like its owner, thought Leo as he sat down in the little black and red vehicle.

"So, this trip to Milan? Did you like it? Is it a nice city?"

"It is, it's not bad at all, something I wasn't

expecting. I suppose like everyone else, I thought it was a big industrial city, but the old town is quite charming."

"So did you meet that Maeva lady? Do you want to talk about it? If not, I'll understand! Just tell me. You know, me too, I think I have things I'd like to understand in this story, I did lose my best friend. I was really close to your mom."

"Yeah, I know. And it doesn't bother me to talk about it, quite the opposite."

They drove out of the airport and were already on the way to Lausanne, making sure they didn't speed because the Swiss authorities were intransigent about that.

"You left because you had a lot of questions, if I remember correctly? Did you get any answers?"

"Sure did! And even more than I was expecting, to tell the truth. I can assure you I heard an incredible story. If all that's true, it's crazy!"

"Really? How come? So this lady wasn't actually your father's mistress?"

"Yes, she was," Leo said. "She was his mistress and now she's even more than that?"

"Meaning?"

Leo didn't know where to start to tell her everything he'd learned about his parents, Maeva, and himself at the same time. While Aline was passing the long line of trucks, he began.

"Okay. I"ll give you the short version. Genetically speaking, that woman is my mother."

"What?"

Aline nearly let go of the steering wheel and put her neck out of joint after an abrupt movement of her head towards Leo.

"You heard correctly. I've got her Italian genes in me. Plus, the first time I saw her it was strange and then I saw my own reflection in the mirror when I was shaving. We've got the same nose."

"How can that be possible? What the heck? How can your father's mistress be your biological mother?

While it was drizzling on Lake Geneva and night was falling on Switzerland, Leo told Aline everything he'd learned in Milan. He told her everything he knew about his father's affair, about his mother's despair about her infertility, plus Maeva's totally ridiculous idea. How she'd convinced his father, how his father had convinced his wife. Then he told her about the famous professor's secret intervention, and once again this unsettling physical resemblance.

Aline, for the first time in her life, didn't say a word. That gave Leo free rein to continue.

"See, I didn't go all this way for nothing! But I still have a little question and I think that since you were her best friend, you could answer it."

"Go ahead. I'll tell you anything I know, I'm not going to hide anything. You have the right to know."

They'd now passed Lausanne and were driving

towards Jougne, getting nearer to France. The windshield wipers were going at full speed as it was now pouring.

Leo looked at her.

"Did my mom have a lover too?" Aline suddenly raised her eyebrows.

"Why are you asking that?"

"That's sort of the impression I had when I was reading her diary and looking at my dad's CD-ROM."

"She said she had an affair in her diary?"

"Not really, but several times she wrote sentences that made me think she did."

"Like what?"

"She wrote stuff like, "*I can't wait to see him*," "*It does me so much good when we see each other*," "*I'm ashamed to be lying to Sacha.*" "*Should I come clean or hide it?*", stuff like that."

"I see."

"Plus each time she wrote *him* or *he* with capital letters. When you do that, it means something."

Suddenly Noemie's best friend burst out laughing, astonishing Leo.

"What? What's so funny?"

"I see what you're getting at Leo and believe me, it has nothing to do with your mom cheating on your dad. I'm sure your mom would never have been able to cheat on him, even if she was hopeless."

"So who was this Him?"

"A shrink!"

"A shrink?"

"Yup, a psychologist. Your mom needed someone to talk to for a couple of months to cope, to help her when nothing was working to have you. Plus she'd told me that your father was totally opposed to the idea of her consulting someone like this. That's why she always did it on the sly, like you would do with a lover."

"I can't believe it," Leo admitted. "And to think that I was totally out of the ballpark here with that. I would have even found it normal for her to have had the temptation, just like my dad."

Aline nodded.

"Just reread those passages and I bet that they'll all match the fact she was seeing a shrink."

While they were driving Leo tried to remember the exact sentences and it did seem to him now that they could have been interpreted differently.

After having driven for over two hours, they were nearing Besancon.

"What are you going to do now?" Aline asked.

"About what?"

"About Maeva of course. If she's the person she says she is, she's important to you, isn't she?"

"I don't know yet. This is all too recent and so enormous. She seemed to be sincere when she said she was ready to play a substitution role for me. But I have to digest all this, things will become clearer as time goes by. Plus I have to take care of Chloe, of our marriage and try to have our own family."

"Ah! Love.." Aline concluded. "It's sometimes tough, but often so beautiful."

Aline dropped him off at home where Chloe was waiting for him.

Chapter 50

Besançon, February 19, 1990

MATERNITY WARD **in Saint-Jacques Hospital**

"IT'S A BOY!" said the midwife, as if it were the very first child she'd helped to be born. "What's his name going to be?"

"Leo," they both said at the same time.

"Do you want to cut the cord?"

Sacha was proud to have been asked to do this task, a unique one in a man's life.

The midwife put the baby on Noemie's bosom: instinctively he looked for and found his mother's breast.

"He's got his father's ears... and his mother's nose!" declared the midwife, with her expert eyes.

Sacha hugged his wife and their tears mingled, running down on the little patch of Leo, their son's, hair.

Chapter 51

Besançon, February, 2015

PIPPO HAD the target in his line of sight, observing it from his huge windshield. He'd have to be quick and reactive.

"Surprise them," he sneered out loud in his cab.

Outside, the sidewalks were still white, frost was still on the windows of the buildings. The few passersby walked with their heads down, beneath a hood, their necks hidden in their shoulders, trying to make sure the wind and cold couldn't get to them. No one seemed to pay attention to this semi with its Italian plates, purring like a huge tomcat in the empty supermarket parking lot.

"Good, the less witnesses, the better things will be," muttered Pippo, taking another sip of *grappa* right from the bottle. He always kept a little stock of miniature bottles of *grappa* in his cab. To warm up. Or to give himself the courage he'd still be needing, though his hatred and his spirit of revenge had already been guiding him for many years now.

He was ready. The night before, he'd checked everything out, first on foot, then in his semi. He'd calculated everything.

It could work. It had to work!

To be honest though, he'd begun checking and following way before yesterday. Way before he'd gone to Besancon.

Years before.

To be honest, since he got out of prison, three years ago, in Milan.

His desire to exact vengeance was at its paroxysm when he'd left the Milan prison, with a sack on his shoulder and despair for his only horizon.

He'd succeeded in finding *her*. She was still as beautiful, perhaps even more so. The saucy little girl he'd known had become a beautiful woman, visibly assuming her femininity and her sex-appeal. The contrast with himself, now overweight, nearly bald with rotten teeth, merely accentuated his bitterness. She was the image of *joie de vivre*; he embodied bile, stench and acidity.

First, he'd thought of attacking her directly. He'd envisaged several scenarios, from easy ones up to complicated ones. He's imaged torturing her, cruel brutality, making her suffer.

As she hadn't wanted to share his life, he'd decided to take hers!

But he wasn't brave enough to carry out any of these macabre plans.

Little by little, the more he spied on her and followed her, the more he was convinced that killing her wouldn't be enough. With this solution he'd probably find himself behind bars once again, but on a one-way trip this time.

Then one day fate knocked on his door and he thought of something different.

She was seeing someone, regularly. A good-looking guy. Though it really didn't seem to him they were lovers. Nonetheless, gestures and attitudes they shared betrayed a type of complicity, they must have been attracted to each other in the past.

Since Pippo got out of prison, he'd had time to spy on them. He'd discovered who this man was, where he lived, what kind of life he had. He could tell by his accent that he was French.

And little by little he was able to retrace this strange couple's past. A few years ago they had been lovers. He was still married and was now a father. Now that he knew all that, he was going to use this info to make her suffer, that woman who was a living ghost of his own past, that woman who was the nightmare of his present.

Because he drove a semi, he often went to France and took advantage of this to finetune his research and confirm his intuitions.

He'd reached the conclusion that taking care of *him* would allow him to reach *her*!

Just killing *her* would have simply closed the file.

But killing *him* would make *her* suffer terribly: she'd know that she was responsible for his death. If he died, she'd be indirectly responsible and she'd suffer until the end of her days.

That was the solution he liked the best for his revenge, his vengeance.

The solution he was now rolling out on this cold winter morning.

His Scania's windshield wipers were chasing away the thin layer of snow on his front window. On his left he was able to see the large black Volvo V60 that was nearing the traffic light. The car was still accelerating, so the light must have been green and his was red.

Pippo let the five-hundred horsepower semi go. The cab shook, the truck coughed, but as it was empty, it quickly picked up speed. His light was still a bright red.

He roared through it.

The Volvo was surprised, it went into a spin on the slippery road where it couldn't stop.

Pippo had just enough time to see the look in the eyes of the passengers, a man and a woman.

A man he knew well now...

The Volvo spun underneath the Scania, between the cab and the trailer and flattened near its gas tank, which was full, just like an accordion.

The whole neighborhood must have heard that explosion, waking up the many inhabitants of Besancon who were still sleeping soundly this Sunday morning.

Pippo's macabre mission was finished.

Chapter 52

Paris, Concorde Lafayette Hotel, 2005

JACQUES SIETHBÜLLER TOOK a deep breath and put a hand on his colleague's shoulder.

"How long have we known each other, Francois... thirty years? You're my friend, at least I hope so."

"Of course I am Jacques!"

"My career is nearly over, who knows, maybe my life too."

"Oh come on, Jacques," N'Gapet protested.

"Let's just say that I'm nearing the finish line then... Francois?"

"Yes?"

"There's something I'd like to tell you."

"Go ahead.

"Thanks. I've been keeping this to myself for

such a long time that I think it's time I got rid of this burden. I knew I could count on you. But hear me out till the end before saying anything, it'll be easier for me."

∽

PARIS, **May, 1989,**

"IT WAS ALREADY PITCH *black when I walked across the little wooded courtyard in front of the hospital. I'd walked quickly and with assurance, so no one would suspect anything had they seen me. People tend to be suspicious when you look like you're wandering around.*

So as I remember, it must have been in the fall, because I could hear the leaves crackling beneath my feet when I went under the weeping willows. I walked straight towards Building C1. It was an old, isolated Haussmann style building, but despite the way it looked, it had sliding glass doors that required a magnetic key card to get in. Of course, as head of the department, I had one.

So no problem for me to gain entry.

Inside, all the lights were out except for the green lights on the emergency exit signs. I also knew that at this time of the night, the building would be deserted. So no one would be there to bother me. I still didn't turn on the lights though and walked down the hall, only guided by those greenish and spectral lights. Like it was almost supernatural.

About thirty feet down the hall was the door I'd been

looking for. It had a digital code. I didn't come here very often, because I didn't need to for my job, but I still knew the code.

I don't know what would have happened if I'd come across a guard? Would he have recognized me? But no, I was all alone in the building.

After keying in the six-figure code, I heard a little click and went into the laboratory, which was nearly dark except for a bunch of little red, green, blue or orange lights, anyway, you know what I'm talking about here Francois! It's strange, this type of lab always makes me think of the kitchen for schools: machines that look like mixers or blending machines, fridges or yogurt machines. But when you think about it, in vitro fecundation is our little recipe. We mix a few things together and create something new! But each time the recipe is only used once. Even though it could technically be reproduced forever, but that's another story.

I WENT RIGHT UP *to the incubator to get the test tube I was interested in.*

My dear friend, I won't tell you all the details that led me to make this secret nocturnal visit, nor the names of the protagonists and their motivations, including mine. But I want you to know that a few days earlier, I had supervised the harvesting of oocytes of one of my patients, a volunteer egg cell donor, and I put a miniscule mark on her test tube so that I could identify it later. See Francois, it was premeditated! There wouldn't be any mitigating circumstances for me in front of the jury!

After looking at about ten tubes in the liquid nitrogen

bath, I finally found the one with the mark on it, the one that had the genes of this donor I knew well and who I'd promised to do something for.

I have to admit here Francois, that I was battling against my professional ethics. Hippocrates' shadow was over me! I was getting ready to commit an irreparable crime: eugenics. I was going to interfere in a process that deontologically had to remain anonymous and random. Ethics and the law forbid me to mix the genes with those of a man who I also knew to create an embryo for another woman: his wife.

I hesitated for many long minutes, holding the test tube, before deciding..."

∽

PARIS, **Concorde Lafayette Hotel, 2005**

"SO WHAT DID YOU DO, JACQUES?" asked Professor N'Gapet, finishing up his glass of champagne.

"I did what I had to do, both as a doctor and as a man."

"Meaning?"

"Well... I put the test tube back where it was at the beginning, and I closed the container."

"So you didn't interfere in the medically assisted procreation process of the couple then?

"No, I didn't. I finally decided to let fate take its course, saying to myself that there would actually be a chance that they'd use this test tube. The honest doctor I've always been won out over the corruptible man who festers in all of us."

"So none of those involved knows the truth?"

"That's right. Neither anyone nor I know the truth about the genes of this man, of these two women and about the child who was born from this strange trio."

"Anyway Jacques, nothing forbids us from thinking that after all fate did choose to mix the sperm of this man with the oocytes contained in the test tube of this not so anonymous donor then? It's a possibility, isn't it?"

"You're right. Only a DNA test could give us the answer. But I don't think that any of the parties, whoever they are, really want that."

The two doctors finished their conversation, toasting each other once again.

"To life, and to its mysteries!"

Epilogue

Above the Alps, July, 2025

THE JET WAS FLYING at thirty thousand feet, south-south-east, from Paris to Milan Malpensa.

"Wow! Daddy, look at the Earth! Is that snow, all that white stuff?"

"Yup, it's the snow that never melts on the peaks of the Alps. Do you realize that right now we're flying even higher than the highest peak of the Alps, Mont-Blanc? Did you learn how high it is at school?"

"Um... I think it's fifteen thousand seven hundred feet?"

"That's about right, I think. Did you know that its height changes over time? When I was at school, they taught me that it was fourteen thousand nine hundred and ninety feet. It increased by…"

"Ten feet!" shouted the little boy sitting between his parents. "Do you think it's an adult now?"

All three of them burst into laughter, like kids in a playground.

"Are you happy to go see *Nonna* Maeva?" asked Leo, running his hand through his son's blond hair.

"Yeah! Really happy! She said she'd make me some Italian ice-cream."

"She's real good at that!" added Chloe, licking her lips.

Then the flight attendant came to serve them their traditional snacks served on Alitalia's medium-haul flights.

"*Nonna* Maeva told me you were going to tell me how you met."

"And *Nonna* Maeva is always right!" replied Leo. "It's important that you understand where you came from, that you know your own personal history, what happened before you were actually born."

"I don't understand anything Daddy!"

"That's normal," sighed Leo. "I was just thinking out loud, talking to myself."

"Isn't it funny that we're talking about that in the plane taking us to Milan?" said Chloe, rescuing him. "Because thirteen years ago your dad and I met in an airport. It was a summer job for me, I was processing tickets and luggage for passengers, you know like they did in Paris when our suitcases disappeared from the conveyor belt, behind those plastic curtains?"

"Yeah, I see. And were you taking a plane, Daddy?"

"Yes, I was. I was going to Crete on vacation and when I was checking in, I saw your mom's beautiful eyes. Because they are beautiful!"

"They look like diamonds!" said Nino. "I have the same ones!"

"Both of you are my little jewels! So we looked at each other and I got lost in her eyes. And you should have heard her voice when she asked for my passport! It's simple, as if she was asking me to marry her! So then we started talking, just like that, at the counter, everyone behind me was starting to get pretty impatient, just like they do as usual in airports. Like they were going to miss their flights, even though the planes are always late! So anyway, we exchanged our phone numbers and said we'd see each other somewhere else than at an airline counter, like have a drink in a bar or something. So there you go! That's how it all started. Seems to be a habit in this family."

"How come?"

Leo was tempted to explain but decided not to.

"I'll tell you all that when you're bigger and you can understand. All I can say now is that you'll probably fall in love with someone who works in the airline industry. Maybe this pretty flight attendant, the one at the back. What do you think, she's cute, isn't she?"

"Come on! She's too old for me," replied Nino.

"Shhh! What if she heard you? She wouldn't like that."

The flight ended with this joyful atmosphere. About forty-five minutes later, they met Maeva in the arrival's hall.

"Nino!" shouted out the woman whose grey hair was in an elegant chignon. "Come to *Nonna*! Give your grandma a big kiss! You ungrateful kids!" she said to Leo and Chloe. "You could at least come see me more often. He's getting so big. Just look at his cute cheeks and his little blond curls."

"But just a second *Nonna*," said Leo, cutting her off as he knew she could wax on for hours when she began talking about her grandson. "It seems to me that as a former Alitalia employee, you've still got good prices and you could come see us more often."

"Did you make me some ice-cream?"

"Tons of vanilla ice-cream!"

All four of them walked out hand-in-hand in Milan's sunny weather.

Report from the Besançon Police Station

Monday, February 16, 2015

Subject: **Accident on a public road**

The accident that took place on Sunday in Besancon in the Saint-Claude district had three victims.

Passengers of the black V60 Volvo were identified as being Mr. Sacha Terebus, sixty years old and his wife, Mrs. Noemie Terebus, née Kapinsky, fifty-six years old.

Sacha Terebus was well-known in the region for his activity as an engineer in the field of nanotechnologies. He was also very active in associations in his district and in Besancon.

Noemie Terebus was a French teacher in the Victor Hugo middle school in Besancon. The daughter of the Russian violinist, Grigor Kapinsky, she was passionate about the French language, her second language.

The third victim of Italian origin, was harder to identity. His semi had Italian license plates and caught fire. His body was partially burned, making it difficult to identify him as his papers were also destroyed.

After an investigation however involving our Italian colleagues with the victim's employer, *Gruppo Pirelli* in Milan, we have reached the conclusion that this man, age sixty approximately, was Filippo Risi.

The Pirelli Group informed us that the driver had delivered his payload of new tires to the Peugeot Facility in Sochaux, though they had no idea what he could have been doing on Sunday, in Besancon. They however added that he had a day off before going back to Milan.

The Italian driver had a low alcohol level in his blood.

There were no known links between the three victims of the accident.

We consequently conclude that it was a simple accident with possible aggravating circumstances concerning the alcoholic content and/or fatigue (lack of vigilance?) of the semi driver. It has also been established that the road was slippery due to snow and ice.

This file has thus been closed.

Also by Nino S. Theveny

[30 seconds before dying](#) (English Version, 2021)

[8 more minutes of sunshine](#) (English Version, 2021)

French Riviera (English Version, 2023)

Into Thin Air (English Version, 2023)

I Want Mommy (English Version, 2023)

Notes

Chapter 8

1. Youth is the teacher for crazy people.
2. The die has been rolled.

Printed in Dunstable, United Kingdom